Lasers in Cutaneous Medicine
and Surgery

LASERS IN CUTANEOUS MEDICINE AND SURGERY

JOHN L. RATZ, M.D.

Staff Physician
Department of Dermatology
The Cleveland Clinic Foundation
Cleveland, Ohio

YEAR BOOK MEDICAL PUBLISHERS, INC.
CHICAGO • LONDON

0   9   8   7   6   5   4   3   2   1

Library of Congress Cataloging-in-Publication Data

Ratz, John Louis.
  Lasers in cutaneous medicine and surgery.

  Includes bibliographies and index.
  1. Skin—Surgery. 2. Argon lasers—Therapeutic use.
3. Carbon dioxide lasers—Therapeutic use. 4. Lasers in surgery. I. Title. [DNLM: 1. Lasers—therapeutic use.
2. Skin—surgery. WR 650 R279L]
RD520.R38 1986   617'.477   85-27137
ISBN 0-8151-7074-2

Sponsoring Editor: David K. Marshall
Manager, Copyediting Services: Frances M. Perveiler
Copyeditor: Deborah Thorp
Production Project Manager: Carol Ennis Coghlan
Proofroom Supervisor: Shirley Taylor

I warmly dedicate this book to those I love:
to SHIRLEY, *my wife;*
KRISTI, T.J., *and* STACIE, *my children;*
and VERONICA, *my mother.*

CONTRIBUTORS

GREGORY T. ABSTEN, M.A.

President, The Laser Forum
Developmental Consultant
Grant Hospital Laser Center
Columbus, Ohio

DAVID B. APFELBERG, M.D., F.A.C.S.

Director, Comprehensive Laser Center
Palo Alto Medical Foundation
Assistant Clinical Professor, Plastic Surgery
Stanford University Medical Center
Stanford, California

PHILIP L. BAILIN, M.D.

Chairman, Department of Dermatology
The Cleveland Clinic Foundation
Cleveland, Ohio

ELIZABETH I. McBURNEY, M.D.

Clinical Associate Professor of Dermatology
Louisiana State University School of Medicine and
Tulane Medical School
Staff Physician
Charity Hospital
New Orleans, Louisiana
Private Practice
Slidell, Louisiana

JOHN A. PARRISH, M.D.

Professor of Dermatology
Harvard Medical School
Director, Wellman Laboratory
Massachusetts General Hospital
Boston, Massachusetts

JOHN L. RATZ, M.D.

Staff Physician
Department of Dermatology
The Cleveland Clinic Foundation
Cleveland, Ohio

CHRISTOPHER R. SHEA, M.D.

Clinical and Research Fellow
Department of Dermatology
Harvard Medical School
Wellman Research Laboratory
Massachusetts General Hospital
Boston, Massachusetts

OON TIAN TAN, M.D.

Instructor, Dermatology
Harvard Medical School
Assistant in Dermatology
Massachusetts General Hospital
Boston, Massachusetts

PREFACE

The birth of laser medicine in the early 1960s was largely due to the hard work and persistence of my friend and colleague Leon Goldman, M.D. We are greatly indebted to him for his foresight, early contributions, and continued work in the area of laser dermatology.

Since the birth of laser dermatology, written material about laser application has been limited mostly to scattered articles appearing in a number of periodical medical publications. Recently, several books covering the areas of laser dermatology and plastic surgery have been published, but with a slightly different approach than that offered by *Lasers in Cutaneous Medicine and Surgery.* Aimed at dermatologic surgeons, plastic surgeons, and those physicians who employ cutaneous surgery in their practices, the goal of *Lasers in Cutaneous Medicine and Surgery* is to offer a very direct and practical approach to the application of both the argon and the carbon dioxide lasers for specific treatable entities. It is presented in a "this is how we do it, and this is what you should expect" type of approach. The observations and comments made are of great import to the physician first embarking on laser surgery.

Before looking at the practical applications of these lasers, however, anyone not well versed in laser physics can acquire reasonable knowledge in this area by means of the first chapter of this book. This material is compiled in an easily understood delivery of an often very difficult subject. The chapter is comprehensive and discusses not only theoretical parameters but also various clinical observations that sometimes refute the theory. These topics are again discussed in the respective chapters on practical application. Even at the time of publication, however, the power densities one uses to achieve the best overall results with both lasers are still a matter of considerable controversy. Such questions may be answered soon, but the answers may actually be unnecessary because of the progress and development of other newer laser systems.

This final area of laser research and development is reviewed in the final chapter in this text. Much of what appears to be possible seems to fit in the realm of 21st-century medicine. It is hoped that this chapter will provoke new thoughts and new ideas for further advancing laser applications in cutaneous medicine and surgery.

It is difficult to compile a timely text in such a rapidly advancing field. This is certainly not possible without the help of many many people. The work on this text is no exception. I would like to thank the contributors to this text and especially their secretaries. I would like to specifically thank Cynthia Wright, R.N., Yvonne Becknell, and Patty Haney for their efforts in helping compile much of the early treatment data for the CO_2 laser. I would also like to thank Nancy Heim from the Cleveland Clinic Foundation art department for her fine work in graphic illustration. Finally, I would like to thank Hope Levitt, my secretary, for her endurance and hard work in helping prepare much of this manuscript.

JOHN L. RATZ, M.D.

CONTENTS

1

LASER BIOPHYSICS FOR
THE PHYSICIAN

GREGORY T. ABSTEN, M.A.

THE PAST DECADE has seen an enormous increase in the use of new technologies in medicine. As one of these new technologies, the laser has already found many applications, and the list is growing. Laser technology will ultimately contribute to a broad and rapid expansion of both diagnostic and treatment procedures.

Experimental work with lasers has brought us to the subatomic realm, by tapping the very forces that hold matter together. This technology is thus not simply another step along the continuum of electronics but an evolution to a higher level. Those physicians who wish to apply state-of-the-art medicine for the maximum benefit of their patients will surely need to be knowledgeable concerning this new and growing technological field.

The purpose of this chapter is to review the subject of biomedical lasers and to provide a basic foundation for learning the practical techniques of laser surgery and for keeping pace with future developments in this area.

LASER PHYSICS

Laser is an acronym for light amplification by stimulated emission of radiation. Laser thus refers to a process by which light waves are amplified and not merely to the device that produces this effect. The process of stimulated emission was first described by Albert Einstein in the early 1900s as an offshoot of his quest to show the inherent singular nature of the four basic forces of the universe. It was not until the late 1950s that Arthur Schawlow and Charles Townes proposed the first practical laser based on Einstein's theories, and Theodore Maimon constructed the first ruby laser in 1960. After the technical development of the laser device, much credit must go to Leon Goldman, a University of Cincinnati dermatologist, for his foresight and continued perseverance in applying this light to the practice of medicine and surgery.

Light is only one small portion of a continuum of electromagnetic energy that goes from cosmic rays to radio waves. Laser radiation is in or near the range of visible light in the electromagnetic spectrum. Radiation is commonly viewed as the high-energy ionizing type of radiation that is associated with x-rays or radiation therapy. But surgical laser radiation is radiant energy at a much longer wavelength; as such, it is not associated with the radiation hazards of x-ray exposure.

Although the exact nature of light is still not understood, it does exhibit characteristics of both discrete particles, or photons, and waves. For purposes of understanding the electromagnetic spectrum and lasers, we shall discuss light primarily in terms of its wave characteristics.

Light Waves

A wave is characterized by four qualities: wavelength (λ), frequency (f), velocity (v), and amplitude (A) (Fig 1–1). The wavelength is the distance between two successive crests. The wavelengths of visible light waves range from about 385 to 760 nm (Fig 1–2). The color of visible light is determined by its wavelength. The chart of the electromagnetic spectrum is organized according to wavelength (Fig 1–3). We usually speak of the wavelength of laser light in terms of

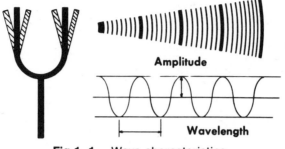

Fig 1–1.—Wave characteristics.

LIGHT PARTICLES

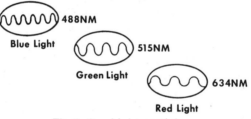

Fig 1–2.—Light particles.

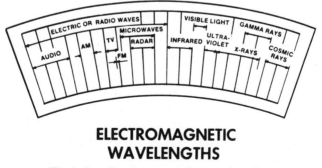

ELECTROMAGNETIC WAVELENGTHS

Fig 1–3.—Electromagnetic wavelengths.

nanometers (nm), and at times in terms of micrometers (μm) or Angström units (Å). The relationships among these units are as follows:

$$1 \ \mu m = 0.001 \ mm \ (10^{-3} \ mm)$$
$$= 1000 \ nm$$
$$= 10,000 \ Å$$

$$1 \ nm = 0.000001 \ mm \ (10^{-6} \ mm)$$
$$= 0.001 \ \mu m$$
$$= 10 \ Å$$

$$1 \ A = 0.0000001 \ mm \ (10^{-7} \ mm)$$
$$= 0.0001 \ \mu m$$
$$= 0.1 \ nm$$

Amplitude refers to the height of the waveform. The frequency of a wave is the number of waves passing a given point per second and is usually expressed in cycles per second, or hertz. Because the velocity of electromagnetic waves is constant at 3×10^8 m/sec (186,000 miles/second), frequency and wavelength are inverse relationships. That is, the shorter the wavelength, the higher the frequency, and vice versa. Since the radiant energy is proportional to the frequency, the shorter wavelengths have more energy. That is why ionizing (x-ray) radiation carries more energy than visible light.

Energy Levels

To understand how a laser works and how its light differs from other light, we must review the basic rules of quantum mechanics.

In an atom, electrons occupy certain discrete levels, or orbits. The higher the energy level of an atom, the farther out will be the orbits of its electrons (Fig 1–4). These electrons are not free to occupy levels between the discrete orbits, so that when the energy level of an atom is changed, electrons must move up or down to the next orbital level. An atom absorbs energy to make this transition upward and emits energy when the transition is downward. The energy is absorbed or emitted as photons, or particles of radiant energy. In the case of lasers, this emitted radiation is in the infrared, ultraviolet, or visible light spectrum.

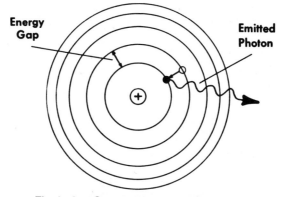

Fig 1–4.—Quantum nature of an atom.

An atom can be excited to a higher energy level by absorbing a photon, but only if the energy of the photon is equal to the energy difference between the orbits. Excitement will not occur if the photon does not possess the same energy (and hence color, wavelength, and frequency).

Ordinarily, an electron's orbit will spontaneously decay from its high-energy state back to its resting base state. This process causes a photon to be emitted spontaneously. When many atoms in a medium undergo spontaneous orbital decay, the photon emissions are out of phase with one another. This spontaneous decay is entirely random, emitting light of many colors and in many directions. This light is known as incoherent light (Fig 1–5). In the laser process,

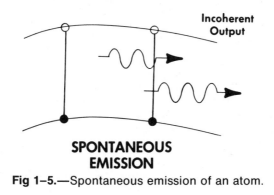

**SPONTANEOUS
EMISSION**

Fig 1–5.—Spontaneous emission of an atom.

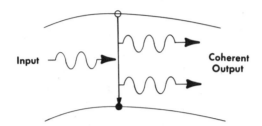

STIMULATED EMISSION
Fig 1–6.—Stimulated emission.

however, an electron in an excited state is stimulated by a photon of precisely the correct energy to cause the atom to undergo orbital decay and emit another, identical photon (Fig 1–6). The end result is that two photons of equal wavelength (or color) leave the atom together in exactly the same direction and perfectly in phase with each other. This light is known as coherent light.

For a medium to possess lasing action, therefore, one of the first requirements is that it have more atoms that are in the higher energy state than atoms that are in the resting level state. This situation is known as *population inversion* of the medium.

Special Qualities of Laser Light

The process of stimulated emission gives rise to the three unique characteristics of laser light as compared with ordinary light: coherence, collimation, and monochromaticity.

Coherence describes the wave patterns of two photons being in phase with one another in both time and space (Fig 1–7). It is analogous to a smooth, even surf breaking on a beach in neatly organized rows. By contrast, the chop produced on the surface of a shallow lake by a multitude of water skiers corresponds to incoherence. When the waves are all in phase, this coherence has an additive effect on their amplitude (see Fig 1–7, A). This additive effect constitutes the beginning of the process of amplification.

Collimation means that the photons do not appreciably diverge from one another as they travel outward. The path of the two photons approaches a perfectly parallel course, so that there is virtually

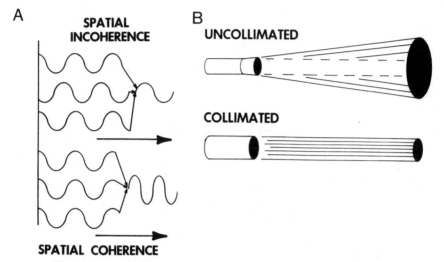

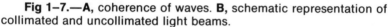

Fig 1–7.—A, coherence of waves. **B,** schematic representation of collimated and uncollimated light beams.

no beam divergence. For our purposes, collimation means that the power level of the beam remains the same no matter how far it is measured from the laser tube. In contrast, the beam of a flashlight diverges increasingly as the object encountered increases in distance from the light source (Fig 1–7, B). With the collimated light of a laser beam, however, 80 to 100 W of light released from the end of the laser tube can be delivered to the surgical field with a minimal loss of power. Owing to the physics of wave optics, collimation also means that the light beam can be focused down to pinpoint spot sizes, a key factor in the surgical application of laser power.

Monochromaticity indicates that the emitted photons are of identical color (or wavelength). Some lasers produce an output that contains more than one wavelength, however. The argon laser, for example, produces outputs primarily at 488 nm (blue) and 515 nm (green). As these outputs occur at discrete points on the spectrum rather than spread over a band, it is not incongruous to speak of the laser as monochromatic. In most types of laser surgery, maintaining the absolute spectral purity of the laser beam is unnecessary. The beam is primarily used for its brute-force thermal effects on tissue, and its color merely indicates how efficiently this thermal transfer is occurring. It is possible to "fine tune" the color of some lasers, if desired.

One area in which the spectral purity of the laser beam is critical is photoradiation therapy, developed by Thomas Dougherty, Ph.D., at Roswell Park in Buffalo, N.Y. James McCaughan, M.D., of the Medical Laser Research Foundation at Grant Hospital, Columbus, Ohio, currently has one of the largest caseloads in this area. In photoradiation therapy, a type of human hematoporphyrin derivative (HHPD) is administered systemically. In about 72 hours, major differences in residual drug levels exist between normal and malignant cells. By itself, the drug is latent, but when activated by specific colors of intense light that a laser may provide, it becomes toxic. The type of laser light used in photoradiation therapy produces no thermal effects and is used solely to initiate phototoxic processes in the cell via the drug. This and other specialized uses of tunable lasers are discussed by Parrish and colleagues in Chapter 4.

LASER DEVICES

A laser device consists of four primary components: an active medium, an excitation mechanism, a feedback mechanism, and an output coupler.

The active medium is the substance that actually exhibits the laser action. A laser is usually named for its active medium. For example, argon is the active medium in the argon laser. The active mediums can be classified into four general groups:

1. Solid
   a. Ruby
   b. Neodymium–yttrium aluminum garnet (Nd-YAG)
2. Gas
   a. Carbon dioxide (CO_2)
   b. Argon/krypton
   c. Helium-neon
3. Liquid: dye lasers
4. Semiconductor

An excitation mechanism is needed to create population inversion in the active medium. The three excitation mechanisms in current use are direct current (200 to 25,000 V), optical pumping (by strobe lamps), and waveguide (by radio frequency or direct current). A waveguide is a means to create and amplify an electromagnetic field. This field, in turn, supplies the energy to create population inversion.

Different mediums have different methods of excitation. Basically, the gas lasers are excited electrically, and the solid-state and liquid lasers are optically pumped. It is possible to use radio frequency to excite a sealed-tube, waveguided CO_2 gas laser, and this method has worked well with miniature, low-power systems. But higher-power CO_2 lasers require flowing gas and direct-current excitation for maximum performance and reliability. Either type of CO_2 laser system simply plugs into existing wall outlets. Most argon and Nd-YAG systems require 208 V or more of electricity and flowing water for cooling.

The feedback mechanism of a laser is the key to amplifying the light produced by stimulated emission. An optical resonator chamber allows oscillation of the light waves back and forth at the speed of light between its ends. Mirrors are used at each end of the resonator chamber to accomplish the reflection (Fig 1–8). Once the resonator chamber sets up a pulsation of light waves back and forth in the chamber, they must get out in order to become functional. One way to do this is to make one of the mirrors partially transmissive, so that the laser beam can "leak out" at that end of the optical resonator. This "window" created by the partially transmissive mirror acts as the output coupler. The light in the optical resonator therefore continues to accumulate in intensity until it is finally able to exit at one end of the chamber.

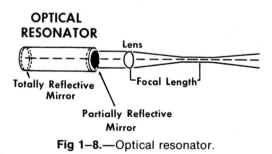

Fig 1–8.—Optical resonator.

Power Density and Spot Size

The power density, or irradiance, of a laser refers to the intensity of the light focused on a particular spot. Power density is the single most important factor in the effective application of any laser. A laser's ability to vaporize, excise, and coagulate various tissues of the body is determined by the power density at which it is set.

Power density is expressed in watts per square centimeter. The surface area of the spot (the spot size) and the total power in watts determine the power density, as follows:

$$\frac{\text{watts} \times 100}{\pi r^2} = \text{watts/cm}^2$$

where r is the radius of the spot (measured in millimeters).

Spot size is a mathematical concept and does not necessarily equal the impact size, which may be manipulated to be smaller or larger than the spot size. While the optical spot size is theoretical, the impact size refers to the actual physical dimensions of the crater or incision. So, although it is a useful measurement, one should not rely overly on the reported spot sizes of different lasers. While power density is a function of spot size and total power in watts, spot size, in turn, is determined by the focal length of the lens, the wavelength of the laser, and the transverse electromagnetic mode (TEM) of the beam.

The smaller the focal length of the lens, the smaller the spot size will be and the more intense the power density will be. On a CO_2 laser with a 400-mm lens the spot size may be 0.8 mm, whereas, a 50-mm lens might produce a 0.1-mm spot size. These particular spot sizes are representative of many common CO_2 surgical lasers and are determined by the size and shape of the beam as it enters the lens. It is possible to modify these lens systems so that spot sizes in the range of 0.025 to 0.05 mm are feasible. These spot sizes in the micrometer range are useful in microvascular welding, otology, ophthalmology, and other areas in which exceptionally small focal spots are required from CO_2 lasers.

The wavelength of the light also limits the degree to which the beam may be focused. The shorter the wavelength, the smaller the spot size, all other factors being equal. It is therefore possible to obtain a much smaller spot size with an argon or Nd-YAG than with a CO_2 laser. The choice of which laser to use for a particular procedure is made according to the specific effects of the laser on tissue and to the delivery mechanism rather than on the basis of this diffraction-limited spot size. For example, the Nd-YAG laser produces a smaller diffraction-limited spot size than the CO_2 laser but is not able to create impact sizes in tissue as small as the CO_2 laser because of its scatter.

The transverse electromagnetic mode (TEM) refers to the distribution of power over the spot area and determines the preciseness of the operative spot size. The most fundamental mode, TEM_{00}, shows an even power distribution over the spot, so that most of the power is at the center. There are no other "hot" or "cold" spots. A graph of the intensity of the beam over an axis of the spot exhibits a gaussian distribution, as shown in Figure 1–9. This mode can produce the smallest spots. Its shape also explains how the impact size can be continuously varied, using time or power, while the spot size remains constant. The spot size of a TEM_{00} beam is the area that contains approximately 86% of the total beam power.

Whenever a laser is passed through an optical fiber, the fundamental mode structure of the beam will be lost. When the power level is not distributed in this fundamental manner, it is said to be in a

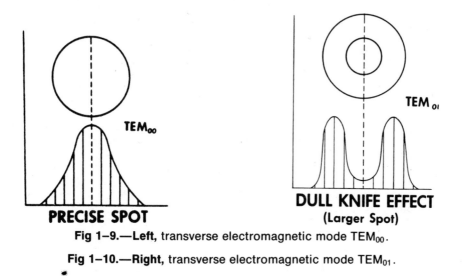

PRECISE SPOT

DULL KNIFE EFFECT
(Larger Spot)

Fig 1–9.—Left, transverse electromagnetic mode TEM_{00}.

Fig 1–10.—Right, transverse electromagnetic mode TEM_{01}.

multimodal distribution. This type of distribution can take many different patterns. A common mode in some commercially available lasers is TEM_{01}, which exhibits a cold spot in the center of the beam (Fig 1–10). This pattern is also called the doughnut mode. The surgical effect of this mode is analogous to cutting with a dull knife, although the defocused beam is sufficient for surface area vaporization at a low power density setting, as we shall see.

Let us compare the relative spot sizes and power requirements of TEM_{00} and TEM_{01} to achieve the same tissue effect. A 400-mm lens with TEM_{00} produces a spot size of 0.8 mm, while a 400-mm lens with TEM_{01} produces a 2-mm spot. Because the power is not equally distributed, the spot is larger with TEM_{01}.

Since power density is a function of both spot size and total power, we can achieve the same power density of 1,900 W/cm^2 by applying either 60 W in a 0.8-mm spot or 10 W in a 0.6-mm spot. Table 1–1 correlates power density to spot size and lens focal length. The biological effect of the laser depends on its calculated power density, not on the power in watts as read from a power meter.

TABLE 1–1.—POWER DENSITY CHART

	SURFACE AREA (πr^2)				
	0.00785 mm	0.03799 mm	0.15896 mm	0.502 mm	3.14 mm
			LENS FOCAL LENGTH		
	50	125	250	340	430
			SPOT SIZE (TEM_{00})		
POWER (WATTS)	0.1 mm	0.22 mm	0.45 mm	0.6 mm	0.8 mm
80	1,019,108	210,560	50,326	15,924	2,548
70	891,720	184,240	44,036	13,933	2,229
60	764,331	157,936	37,745	11,952	1,910
50	636,943	131,613	31,454	9,960	1,592
40	509,554	105,290	25,164	7,968	1,273
30	382,165	78,968	18,872	5,976	955
20	254,777	52,645	12,582	3,984	637
10	127,388	26,322	6,291	1,922	318
5	63,694	13,161	3,195	996	159

The power density, or irradiance, is a static measurement that does not account for the influence of time. Dosage of the laser beam, which accounts for time, is reported in joules. The number of watts of power multiplied by the delivery time equals the number of joules. For example, 1 W × 1 second = 1 joule; 10 W × 0.1 second = 1 joule. This measure expresses the total dosage but does not describe how concentrated the dosage is.

Fluence combines the concepts of spot brightness and dosage. It is measured in joules per square centimeter. This measure describes the irradiance of the spot as well as the dosage (in joules) delivered within this area. Total incident energy is the cumulative energy delivered to the target site during treatment. Fluence helps conceptualize the total tissue effect of the beam. Obviously, 10 joules/cm² will create more of a tissue effect than 1 joule/cm², since 10 joules/cm² is more concentrated than 1 joule/cm².

The optimum power density for laser ablation of tissue is the highest value that can be safely controlled by the surgeon. Use of the highest possible power density restricts the damage to healthy tissue in the vicinity of the impact by limiting the time of exposure of the beam. When the power density is greater than about 100 W/cm², the amount of tissue damage is proportional to the duration of application of the beam, not to the total power (or wattage). This relationship does not hold for a power density less than 100 W/cm², because it is considered ineffectual.

When a laser of low total power is set at a high power density, the beam is in the focused, or cutting, mode. The laser can be used in this mode to vaporize small spots. In order to debulk and vaporize larger volumes of tissue, however, the spot must be broadened to perhaps the size of a pencil eraser. This defocusing allows for smoother, more uniform vaporization of tissue but requires that higher total power be applied in order to compensate for the dilution of power density. Although it is possible to use the pinpoint spot size of a lower power laser to vaporize a mass, this technique creates uneven ridges, furrows, and bleeding and is generally unsatisfactory for debulking procedures. In dermatologic laser practice, however, the current trend has been to shift to lower total power applications to achieve better cosmetic results. With the advent of computer laser scanners for CO_2 lasers, it is now possible to use a higher power density on a fast scan rate to achieve maximum precision and uniformity. Superpulsed and similar modes will provide for further precision. These innovations are discussed in subsequent sections of this chapter.

Power density is the single most important factor when choosing laser apparatus. The higher the power capability of the laser, the greater are its applications and flexibility in performing surgical procedures. In regard to particular procedures, however, power density is a useful but relative concept. Although it is helpful to begin by learning a few rule-of-thumb power densities for use during certain procedures, the surgeon should not become dependent on these numbers for day-to-day practice. Laser surgery requires visual judgment and relative decisions, based on the current situation. At any moment in a particular procedure, the surgeon may decide that the desired effect is either a little more or a little less than the effect being produced by the current laser settings and must be able to make adjustments accordingly. The surgeon must, above all, be able to control the effects of the beam. The maximum precision of a CO_2 laser is achieved by using the *highest power density* one can control.

TISSUE INTERACTION AND BEAM DELIVERY

Each type of laser exhibits differing biological effects and is therefore useful for different applications. The three primary types of lasers used for surgery (CO_2, argon, and Nd-YAG) are not directly competitive; they are complementary. The surgical effect of any of these lasers depends on the manner in which the beam distributes its heat. The CO_2 laser boils the water at a small point. It is used primarily to cut and vaporize. The Nd-YAG laser coagulates protein in a larger volume. The argon laser is also a coagulator but is more pigment-sensitive and of lower total power.

The nature of the interaction between laser light and biological tissue can be described in terms of reflection, transmission, scattering, and absorption (Figs 1−11 and 1−12). In order for the light to exert its effect upon tissue, it has to be absorbed. If it is reflected from or transmitted through the tissue, no effect will occur. If the light is scattered, it will be absorbed over a larger area, so that its effects will be more diffuse. A thorough understanding of these four

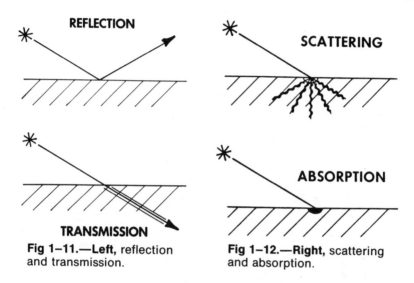

Fig 1–11.—Left, reflection and transmission.

Fig 1–12.—Right, scattering and absorption.

characteristics of the interaction of light with tissue is necessary before the surgeon can select the most appropriate laser system for a particular application.

Regardless of which laser system is used for a surgical application, its effects may be broadly categorized as follows:

1. Coagulation
   a. Necrosis
   b. Hemostasis
2. Vaporization
   a. Cutting
   b. Debulking (evaporating or sublimating tissue)
3. Sonic: membrane disruption

The laser is used for its thermal effect on tissue and the color of the laser beam only determines how efficiently this thermal transfer occurs in different tissue. When it is used to cut or sublimate tissue, the laser actually produces its effect by vaporizing cells. The mechanism of vaporization relies on rapid heat transfer from the beam to the cell. First, the cellular water is superheated to perhaps several hundred degrees past the boiling point of water. This superheating

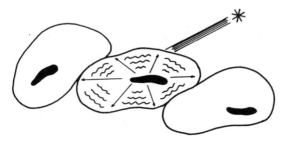

Fig 1–13.—Absorption of energy within the cells.

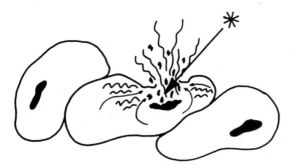

Fig 1–14.—Vaporization and resulting laser plume.

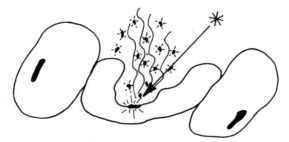

Fig 1–15.—Carbonization of particle fragments.

causes both complete destruction of all cellular proteins and an immense pressure build-up within the cell (Fig 1–13). The rapid rise in intracellular temperature and pressure causes an explosion of the cell, throwing off steam and cellular debris (Fig 1–14). The steam and debris rising from the impact site are seen as the laser plume. This plume remains in the path of the laser beam, and the particle fragments flash white hot as they are carbonized (Fig 1–15).

TYPES OF LASERS

Carbon Dioxide Laser

The carbon dioxide (CO_2) laser has been the primary instrument for laser surgery. The absorption of its middle-infrared output of 10,600 nm (10.6 μm) in biological tissue is independent of tissue color, unlike the argon laser, and its minimization of tissue damage with virtually no scattering differentiates it from the Nd-YAG laser. This high degree of absorption in soft tissue with limited lateral damage is what makes the CO_2 laser a precise surgical instrument for use in vaporizing tissue. Because of its ability to control bleeding and its precision, this laser has been advantageous in Mohs' surgery. Furthermore, the CO_2 laser provides the necessary precision to weld arteries for microsurgery and to anastomose small vessels and nerves. The present use of lasers in dermatologic surgery is nearly equally divided between CO_2 and argon lasers.

In this section, we shall discuss how to manipulate the laser through either a handpiece or a microscope. Even though this discussion will be oriented toward the CO_2 laser, many of these same principles are applicable to all lasers.

The depth of the incision is determined by both the power density and the duration of application (the sweep speed). The feel for controlling the depth of the incision is developed by practice. It is important to maintain a slight tension across the incision line when cutting with the laser.

Laser incisions are considerably less bloody than cold steel incisions. The black char that forms at the edges of the incision is entirely superficial and can be irrigated away. The lateral zone of damage for the CO_2 laser extends less than 0.5 mm from the incision, compared to 4 to 5 mm for the Nd-YAG laser and 5 to 10 mm for electrocautery. Owing to the precise localization of the effects of the CO_2 laser beam, as well as to the sealing effects of the beam, the surrounding tissue exhibits minimal edema, scarring, or stenosis.

Even though progress in the depth of the incision can be seen, once the beam has penetrated the tissue or membrane it instantly travels on to whatever tissue is behind it. For this reason, some type of backstop is needed to prevent damage to the surrounding tissues. Wet sponges or cottonoids are most commonly used for general packing and protection, while quartz rods are used as backstops for very fine dissections.

The CO_2 laser can be applied either with a handpiece or through a micromanipulator attached to a microscope. The transmission of the CO_2 laser through an operative microscope is an excellent technique, because it enables the operator to control the beam precisely and because it enhances visibility in a limited surgical field. A fiberoptic system has also been developed, but it is not yet commercially available to surgeons. Such a system is already in use, however, with the Nd-YAG and argon lasers.

The beam can be manipulated as a surgical tool by adjusting both the power setting of the machine and the spot size. Remember that the CO_2 laser performs with the following order of suitability: cutting, evaporating, and coagulating. When it is used to cut or evaporate tissue, the best approach is to employ the highest power one can safely control. The use of high power localizes the thermal damage to the impact site, thus minimizing the effect on the surrounding tissues. When a CO_2 laser is used to debulk tissue or to coagulate large vessels, the spot size is broadened and the power is increased to compensate. As one's experience grows with the surgical laser, one is able to use higher and higher powers safely. After several months' to a year's experience with the laser, the surgeon may feel comfortable using power levels that are more than double those used initially. Practice is the only way to develop a feel for what a surgical laser can do. This experience can best be initiated through a laser surgery course that includes both theory and hands-on work.

The spot size of the laser beam is adjusted by moving the lens farther from or nearer to the tissue. When the handheld technique is used, manipulation of the spot size is analogous to using a magnify-

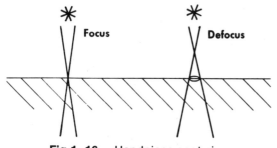

Fig 1–16.—Handpiece spot size.

ing glass. As the lens moves toward the target, the spot reaches its smallest size. In this position, the beam has the highest power density and produces the greatest tissue effects. This "focused" position is primarily used for cutting. By pulling the lens away slightly, one can dampen the tissue effect to produce tissue vaporization or, at a lower power or larger spot size, coagulation (Fig 1–16).

When the laser is used with a microscope, the manipulation is slightly different. The working distance from the tissue is dictated by the objective lens of the microscope. To use the laser through a microscope to cut or vaporize small areas, the spot needs to be at its smallest size, and the highest power density must be used. In order to achieve this setting, the laser lens must match the microscope objective lens; for example, a 300-mm objective lens calls for a 300-mm laser lens. The spot size is then changed by changing the laser lens. When adjusting the laser lens, one need not keep looking at the millimeter labels on the lens. The differences in clarity of the spot can be easily seen. The beam is manually directed by a joystick (Fig 1–17). On devices equipped with variable spot size control, a laser lens is inserted to match the focal length of the objective lens. Once the appropriate laser lens is inserted, the spot size can be varied continuously with a twist control.

Prefocus, or deep focus, means that the laser lens is of a longer focal length than the objective lens of the microscope. Focusing the laser lens will therefore cause the laser spot to be focused at a point below the surface of the target tissue (Fig 1–18). The laser spot will thus be larger on the surface of the target tissue than if it were in focus. The prefocused mode can be used for debulking tissue and, at lower powers, for coagulating vessels. Because the laser focus is

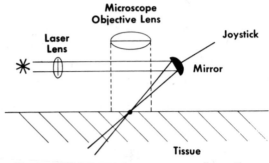

Fig 1–17.—Laser-microscope configuration.

beneath the surface of the target tissue, the surgeon must remain acutely aware of the structures located behind the point of impact. If a prefocused laser is fired in the continuous mode over the same spot, it will burn hotter and faster as it goes deeper, because of the underlying focal point. Similarly, if the surgeon is cutting a tumor remnant overlying a delicate structure such as an artery using a prefocused beam, it is possible to punch a hole in the vessel. In this situation, however, it is also possible to punch a hole in the focused mode. Therefore, except for its use at higher powers or with very proximate delicate structures, the prefocused mode is ordinarily satisfactory for evaporating tissue and coagulating vessels. Remember that with a CO_2 laser you are lasing only what you are seeing. The laser in the prefocused mode will not lase the underlying tissue

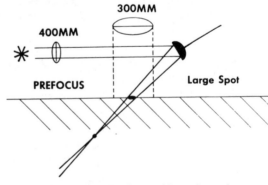

Fig 1–18.—Prefocus (deep focus).

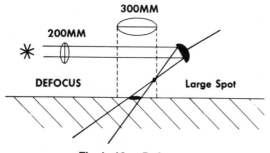

Fig 1–19.—Defocus.

until it vaporizes the tissue above it. In contrast, the Nd-YAG laser can cause coagulation of underlying tissue that is not in the surgeon's view.

The defocused position can be used in much the same way as the prefocused position, except that the focal point of the laser is now above the surface of the target tissue, rather than below it (Fig 1–19). Thus, when the laser in the defocused position is fired in the continuous mode over the same spot, it will burn cooler and slower as it gets deeper, because the spot will spread. When used in the pulsed mode (described in the next paragraph), it may be impossible to tell the difference between the defocused and the prefocused position. Prefocus and defocus are not applicable to a system with variable spot size control, although the concepts are still important for the surgeon to understand.

Another very useful tool for manipulating the tissue effects of the beam is pulsing. Even though the foot pedal can be pumped when the laser is in the continuous mode, the amount of control that is possible with pumping is negligible compared to that of an electronic pulsing mechanism. Decreasing the pulse time has an equivalent effect to decreasing the power settings. For example, the biological effect of 10 W at a 0.2-second pulse is similar to the effect of 20 W at a 0.1-second pulse. As we already mentioned, the term *joules* is used to describe the dosage of the beam on tissue and is the product of the power in watts and the delivery time. This relationship explains why manipulating the duration of the pulses is equivalent to changing the power setting. The power outputs of lasers that are used exclusively or primarily in the pulsed mode, such as

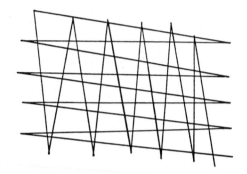

Fig 1–20.—Crisscross pattern for vaporization.

the argon and Nd-YAG lasers, may therefore be expressed in joules or millijoules.

Another way to manipulate the duration of the impact is to wiggle the spot back and forth quickly over the tissue, controlling the movement by hand or by computer. A focused spot at a lower power setting can be used to make a slow incision. If this same focused spot is then wiggled around quickly, it can be used to evaporate tissue. Moved even more quickly, the spot can be used to coagulate vessels and to achieve hemostasis in an area of small bleeders. In this way, the surgeon can obtain several different effects without having to take the time to change the spot size. When evaporating large areas or coagulating an entire field, the spot must be moved back and forth quickly in a crisscross pattern (Fig 1–20).

A microprocessor-controlled CO_2 laser scanner is now available that can be easily programmed to lase any irregular area or line. The surgeon then steps on the laser pedal and the unit automatically and uniformly lases the area. This programming frees up one of the surgeon's hands and allows for a greater degree of uniformity in debulking tissues such as cervical tissue or cranial tumors or in performing dermabrasion.

CUTTING—When the beam is used for cutting, the spot is focused on the tissue. With the laser beam in the focused mode, its effect is precise, and damage is localized. The ability of the beam to seal blood vessels and lymphatic vessels as it cuts creates a dry surgical field that makes many procedures easier and quicker.

The depth of cut is determined by the power density and duration of exposure. The higher the power density applied and the slower the spot is swept across an incision, the deeper the beam will cut. The surgeon can only develop a feel for this technique through practice. In the surgeon's initial laser experiences, the lack of tactile feedback is especially problematic, since this feedback is helpful in gauging the depth of cutting. With experience, the surgeon will be able to increase the power density. Protecting the adjacent tissue also allows for increased speed and decreased risk to the patient.

Incisions made with the laser heal in much the same way as incisions made with a surgical scalpel. Histologically, the scars are identical at 20 to 30 days, even though the order of healing mechanisms is slightly altered. Laser incisions may undergo more rapid reepithelialization, but their tensile strength is less than that of scalpel incisions until 30 to 40 days, when they become identical. In practice, many surgeons say they see no clinical difference between the two wounds after about one week. Skin incisions should be made with a laser only in cases in which the special characteristics of the laser are required.

EVAPORATION—The evaporation (sublimation) of tissue can be performed with the laser in the prefocused or defocused mode. Small areas can be evaporated with a focused spot, but larger areas tend to get ridges and furrows in them if evaporated in this manner. Evaporation is useful in debulking tumors or in removing tissue from delicate structures precisely, one cell layer at a time. Ablative lesions may also be produced with the defocused beam.

Bone and cartilage, because they contain relatively little water, evaporate differently than soft tissue. Bone has a tendency to conduct heat away from the impact site to adjacent tissues. To protect these tissues and limit the thermal damage, a superpulse mode is preferred. This mode appears to produce a continuous beam, but the beam is actually turning on and off about 1,000 times per second, with peak powers up to 500 W on each spike. This pulsing allows a "cooler" cutting of the bone or cartilage. Bone may also need to be irrigated continuously to prevent flaming. The peak power of all laser units that possess the superpulse mode may be varied by the power control on the unit. In addition, some units are equipped with a variable pulse width and rate in the superpulse mode; such features are interesting from an engineering standpoint but offer no additional clinical value.

COAGULATION—While the CO_2 laser instantly coagulates vessels up to 0.5 mm in diameter as it cuts, it is necessary to defocus the spot to coagulate larger vessels. With a defocused beam, vessels up to 2 mm in diameter can be coagulated. Laser evaporation can continue in a bloody field by the use of constant suction. Passing through standing blood with the CO_2 laser only makes a black, sticky coagulum, with continued bleeding underneath. The bloodier the target tissue to be debulked, the higher the power density and wattage and the broader the spot size required for adequate vaporization. Metastases of the liver, for instance, require 70 to 80 W of continuous power at broad spot sizes.

Larger veins, 2 to 5 mm in diameter, may be coagulated with the CO_2 laser and then cut. A defocused beam is first moved slowly over the vessel. The effect is to shrink the vessel so much that its lumen is obliterated. The beam is then switched to the focused mode and the vessel is cut.

Coagulation via argon and Nd-YAG lasers is their natural effect and requires little additional manipulation.

SAFETY MEASURES—Although the CO_2 laser cannot penetrate the eye to the retina, it can still cause corneal and scleral burns. For this reason, protective glasses are required. Ordinary glass or plastic correctional glasses are satisfactory for this purpose, and clear plastic safety glasses are also available. Hard contact lenses will stop the beam but cannot prevent burning, as the lens is in direct contact with the cornea.

Argon Laser

The first major medical application of lasers was the use of the argon laser in the treatment of diabetic retinopathy in 1965. Since that time, and with extensive experience, the argon laser photocoagulator has become the treatment of choice for this retinal disorder. Dermatologic disorders are the other major application of argon laser therapy.

Argon lasers produce a visible blue-green light, with wavelengths at 488 and 515 nm, that is easily transmitted through clear, aqueous tissues. Certain tissue pigments, such as melanin and hemoglobin, absorb argon laser light very effectively. When low levels of this blue-green light interact with highly pigmented tissues, the result is a sufficient level of localized heat generation to make the argon laser a highly effective coagulator. This principle of selective absorption is used to photocoagulate pigmented lesions, such as port-wine hemangiomas and telangiectasias. The argon beam passes through the overlying skin without substantial absorption and reaches the pigmented layer of the lesion, causing protein coagulation in this layer. After the treatment, gradual blanching of the laser-coagulated area occurs over several months. CO_2 lasers are also used extensively in these dermatologic lesions.

When the argon beam is focused to a very small spot (or when the total power is increased sufficiently), its power density is high enough to result in vaporization of the target tissue.

The argon laser can be transmitted through fiberoptics that are only a fraction of a millimeter in diameter. This property makes it possible to use the argon laser through flexible scopes. The beam is transmitted through fibers that are attached to a handpiece that includes a lens system. This technique enhances the use of the argon laser in dermatology.

The micromanipulator for these lasers includes an internal shutter that protects the user when the laser is fired. If the argon laser is used without a microscope, however, special glasses are required.

Argon lasers are typically available in 4- to 10-W units that are adequate for dermatologic applications. Unlike the CO_2 systems, most of these lasers do have special power and plumbing requirements that would necessitate advanced planning for installation.

A system similar to the argon laser is now becoming available. This system makes use of a frequency-doubled Nd-YAG laser that produces light at a wavelength of 532 nm. Higher peak powers are available with this system, and the wavelength may offer advantages in some areas of selective absorption. It will not replace the use of other wavelengths, however.

Nd-YAG Laser

The laser that is best suited for primary coagulative therapy is the neodymium–yttrium-aluminum-garnet (Nd-YAG) laser. Although not nearly as precise as the CO_2 laser, it will coagulate vessels up to about 4 mm in diameter (and larger, with manipulation). The argon laser has also been used to coagulate tissue (e.g., gastrointestinal tract "bleeders"), but its effects are primarily on the hemoglobin and not on the vessel walls.

The Nd-YAG is a solid crystal that is stimulated to emit laser light in the near-infrared region, at a wavelength of 1,060 nm. Nd-YAG laser units are capable of power levels from 15 to 100 W. The laser beam is transmitted to the target tissue through a fiberoptic system.

Because the beam can be transmitted through clear liquids, it can be used in the eye or other water-filled cavities, such as the bladder. Its absorption by tissue is not as color-dependent as the argon laser, so that the Nd-YAG beam is absorbed by almost any tissue that is not clear. The darker the tissue, the greater the absorption.

The physical characteristic that differentiates this laser from the other types is its high degree of scattering on impacting tissue. Focusing an Nd-YAG laser to spot sizes of much less than 2 mm may prove to be of no benefit, because of this high scatter once it impacts soft tissue. The zone of damage produced by an impact is not limited, as it is with the CO_2 laser. A homogeneous zone of thermal coagulation and necrosis may extend 4 mm from the impact site, and precise control is not feasible. Furthermore, it is possible to cause full-thickness injury, necrosis, and sloughing of tissues such as vessels, nerves, and cortex if appropriate precautions (i.e., adjustments in power setting, spot size, and duration of impact) are not taken. These characteristics make the Nd-YAG laser an excellent tool for tissue coagulation, but a very crude tool for the precise control of cutting and for avoiding tissue damage.

The tissue effects of the Nd-YAG laser are complementary to those of the CO_2 laser. It primarily coagulates, can vaporize at sufficiently high power densities, but cuts only crudely and with great difficulty. For this reason, the Nd-YAG laser is used in conjunction with the CO_2 laser in many instances, rather than alone. By using the Nd-YAG laser to coagulate, then using the CO_2 laser to vaporize, large bloody tumors may be removed more easily and in less time than with the CO_2 laser alone.

Although it is possible to combine both lasers in a single unit, a combined unit usually does not prove to be advantageous, since most operating rooms must share equipment among the different specialties. Scheduling conflicts may severely limit the versatility of a combined unit, in that most situations will require the use of one or the other laser. The coupling of separate CO_2 and Nd-YAG laser units may still be achieved when desired, however, by means of various terminal delivery devices. If the lasers are used by one individual or team exclusively, so that scheduling conflicts are not a consideration, the combined unit does offer the advantage of reducing the clutter of two separate machines in the operating room. It can also be used to advantage as an additional laser, rather than as a substitute for the primary CO_2 and Nd-YAG units. As a second laser, the combined unit would provide increased flexibility in scheduling.

It is important to understand that the type of Nd-YAG laser used for surgical procedures is totally different from the type of Nd-YAG laser used by ophthalmologists. The purchase of an ophthalmic Nd-YAG laser unit will not satisfy the requirements of the other specialties, and vice versa. The ophthalmic Nd-YAG laser uses Q-switching or mode locking to create shock wave effects in a spark 50 μm in diameter. This action snaps apart membranes in the posterior capsule of the eye. The effect is sonic and is entirely nonthermal. By contrast, surgical Nd-YAG lasers, even in the pulsed mode, operate as a continuous-wave beam and produce entirely thermal effects. Surgical Nd-YAG lasers also have special power and plumbing requirements. Specially colored safety glasses must be worn. Alternatively, filters may be placed on endoscopes to protect the user.

Outside of its use in ophthalmic surgery, the most common applications of the Nd-YAG laser at present in the United States are in tumor ablation and in the treatment of acute gastrointestinal tract hemorrhage. The goal in controlling hemorrhage is to cause tissue coagulation around the vessel in order to stop the bleeding, rather than coagulating only the hemoglobin, as the argon laser does. The Nd-YAG laser has also been used to open esophageal stenoses for which conventional techniques are not suitable. Neurosurgeons use the Nd-YAG laser for tumor coagulation because of its excellent coagulative abilities and diffuse vaporizing effects.

The Nd-YAG laser is also being used in other specialty areas. Urologists are using this laser via fibers through the cytoscope for tumor vaporization in the bladder. Treatment of urethral strictures with the Nd-YAG laser is also being investigated. Gynecologists use the Nd-YAG laser to vaporize and coagulate the endometrium in the treatment of menorrhagia. Because of its deep penetration, this method may also carry over into the treatment of condylomata. Its use in the laparoscopic treatment of endometriosis is being investigated. Thoracic surgeons and pulmonary specialists are using the Nd-YAG laser via fibers through the biopsy channel of flexible or rigid bronchoscopes. By this method, the laser can then be used in palliative procedures to coagulate endotracheal and endobronchial obstructions.

In the near future, low-power Nd-YAG lasers may see use in the treatment of pain, in tissue welding, and in intravascular procedures to open blocked arteries. The mid-1980s should see a dramatic increase in the use and medical applications of these lasers.

CONCLUSION

The principle advantages of laser surgery are (1) no-touch technique, (2) dry surgical field, (3) reduced blood loss, (4) reduced edema, (5) limited fibrosis and stenosis, (6) no interference with monitoring equipment, (7) potential elimination of residual neoplastic cells, with reduction in recurrences and spread, (8) increased precision, (9) elimination of instruments in field, (10) reduced postoperative pain (in some procedures), and (11) sterile operative site.

In the next few years, the largest area of technological growth will be in the delivery systems for lasers rather than in the lasers themselves. Research groups are currently working on a fiber for the 10.6 μm CO_2 lasers, and systems using this technology may be available by the end of 1985. Endoscopic couplers are an exciting prospect. These couplers allow simultaneous delivery and observation of the laser beam through bronchoscopes, laparoscopes, arthroscopes, gastroscopes, and colonoscopes. As new techniques and instruments, including fiberoptics, are developed to aid in the delivery of lasers to various surgical sites, the field of laser surgery will expand. Before long, even such seemingly farfetched notions as coronary artery surgery on an outpatient basis may become a reality. The laser is an exciting and powerful tool that has already proved its value in many clinical applications. Its future in medicine is bright.

BIBLIOGRAPHY

Abela, G. S., et al. Effects of carbon dioxide, Nd:Yag and argon laser radiation on coronary atheromatous plaques. *Am. J. Cardiol.* 50:1199–1205, 1982.

Anderson, R.; Jaenicke, K.; and Parrish, J. Mechanisms of selective vascular changes caused by dye lasers. *Lasers Surg. Med.* 3(3), 1983.

Andrews, A., and Polanyi, T., eds. *Microscopic and endoscopic surgery with the CO₂ laser.* Boston: John Wright, 1982.

Apfelberg, D., et al. Histology of port wine stains following argon laser therapy. *Br. J. Plast. Surg.* 32:232–237, 1979.

Ben-Bassat, M.; Ben-Bassat, M.; and Kaplan, I. A study of the ultrastructural features of the cut margin of skin and mucous membrane specimens excised by CO_2 laser. *J. Surg. Res.* 21:77–84, 1976.

Bennett, C., ed. *Technos-Lasers* 1(1), 1982.

Bischko, J. Use of the laser beam in acupuncture. *International Journal of Acupuncture and Electro-Therapeutic Research* 5:29–40, 1980.

Boraiko, A. The laser. *National Geographic* 165(3):335–363, 1984.

Caulfield, J. The wonder of holography. *National Geographic* 165(3):365–377, 1984.

Dew, D., and Lo, H. CO_2 laser microsurgical repair of soft tissue: preliminary observations. Presented at the Third Annual Meeting of the American Society for Laser Medicine and Surgery, January 1983, New Orleans.

Einstein, A. *Ideas and Opinions.* New York: Bonanza Books.

Fisher, J. The power density of a surgical laser beam: its meaning and measurement. *Lasers Surg. Med.* 2(4):301–315, 1983.

Fuller, T. A. The physics of surgical lasers. *Lasers Surg. Med.* 1980.

Goldrath, M.; Fuller, T.; and Segel, S. Laser photovaporization of endometrium for the treatment of menorrhagia. *Am. J. Obstet. Gynecol.* 140:14, 1981.

Gore, R. The once and future universe. *National Geographic* 163(6):704–749, 1983.

Green, D., and Cohen, M. Laser interferometry in the evaluation of potential macular function in the presence of opacities in the ocular media. *Trans. Am. Acad. Ophthalmol. Otolaryngol.* 75:629–637, 1971.

Hall, R. R. The healing of tissues incised by a CO_2 laser. *Br. J. Surg.* 58(3):222, 1971.

Hallmark, C. Quantum mechanics. In *Lasers, the light fantastic.* Blue Ridge Summit, Pa.: Tab Books, 1979.

Jain, K. Sutureless microvascular anastomosis using a Nd:Yag laser. *J. Microsurgery* 1:436–439, 1980.

Kroetlinger, M. On the use of the laser in acupuncture. *International Journal Acupuncture and Electro-Therapeutic Research* 5:297–311, 1980.

L'Esperance, F., Jr. An ophthalmic argon laser photocoagulator system: design, construction, and laboratory investigation. *Trans. Am. Ophthalmol. Soc.* 66:827–994, 1968.

Luxon, J. *Applied laser optics.* Toledo: Laser Institute of America, 1983.

Maimon, T. Stimulated optical radiation in ruby. *Nature* 187:493, 1960.

Marchesini, R., et al. Thermal effects of the Nd:Yag laser irradiation: thermographic results. Presented at the Third Annual Meeting of the American Society for Laser Medicine and Surgery, January 1983, New Orleans.

McCaughan, J., et al. Hematoporphyrin derivative and photoradiation therapy of malignant tumors. *Lasers Surg. Med.* 3(3), 1983.

Moritz, A. Studies of thermal energy. III. The pathology and pathogenesis of cutaneous burns: an experimental study. *Am. J. Pathol.* 23:915–927, 1947.

Naisbitt, J. From an industrial society to an information society. In *Megatrends.* New York: Warner Books, 1984.

Norris, C., and Mullarky, B. Experimental skin incision made with the CO_2 laser. *Laryngoscope* 92(4):416–419, 1982.

Polanyi, T. Physics of surgery with the CO_2 laser. In *Microscopic and endoscopic surgery with the CO_2 laser,* ed. A. Andrews and T. Polanyi. Boston: John Wright, 1982.

Tilley, D., and Thumm, W. *Physics.* Philippines: Cummings, 1974.

Verschueren, R. Tissue reaction to the CO_2 laser in general. In *Microscopic and endoscopic surgery with the CO_2 laser,* ed. A. Andrews and T. Polanyi. Boston: John Wright, 1982.

2

USE OF THE ARGON LASER IN DERMATOLOGIC SURGERY

David B. Apfelberg, M.D., F.A.C.S.

Elizabeth McBurney, M.D.

THE UNIQUE and powerful photocoagulation of the argon laser has proved highly valuable in the treatment of an ever-expanding variety of cutaneous lesions. Initial successful management of cutaneous vascular lesions such as port-wine hemangiomas, capillary/cavernous hemangiomas, and telangiectasias has now been extended to many other clinical areas. This chapter summarizes the argon laser treatment of cutaneous vascular abnormalities, tattoos, inflammatory lesions, and a variety of other miscellaneous benign skin lesions.

MATERIALS AND METHODS

The argon laser (Cooper Lasersonics Model 770 or Coherent Radiation Dermatologic Model 1000) used in this clinical work produces intense light in the blue-green combination spectrum at frequencies of 488 and 515 nm. The spot (or aperture) size used varies between 0.2 and 5.0 mm. More precise laser injury is desirable for single or small lesions (such as telangiectasias), while larger, broader lesions with greater area (such as port-wine hemangiomas) may be covered more rapidly by the larger spot size. The power range needed is less for the lighter lesions and greater for the darker lesions, varying between 1.0 and 2.5 W. As a general rule, one uses the minimum amount of power necessary for clinical blanching or vaporization but insufficient to produce scars. The pulse duration most frequently used is 0.2 seconds, but the duration can be varied up to 20 seconds of continuous exposure time for greater concentration of laser power in hypertrophic, spongy, and thick hemangiomas. The choice of continuous vs. pulsed mode often depends on user preference. In either case, the laser stylus is hand held at a distance of 2 to 4 cm perpendicularly to the skin surface and is advanced progressively across the surface of the lesion at a set pace (more rapid with continuous mode, slower for pulsed mode). The pace is set according to the desired clinical effect; for example, hemangiomas require blanching, while tattoos call for vaporization. Total exposure averages 100 to 125 joules/cm^2 of treatment area.

Exposing the skin to one or several argon laser pulses causes a sensation of moderate warmth and discomfort at the treated site. Small lesions can and should be treated without local anesthesia, since injection of an anesthetic can obliterate small vessels and make the delineation of the lesion difficult. For larger lesions or areas (e.g., in port-wine hemangiomas) 2% lidocaine hydrochloride without epinephrine is used for local anesthesia.

Orange safety goggles are worn by all present in the laser operating rooms, and reflective jewelry is removed. Appropriate signs are placed on doors to warn all entering personnel that the laser is in operation, and precautions should be taken to prohibit unauthorized entry. For protection of the patient's eyes during treatment of eyelid lesions, the cornea is anesthetized with 0.05% proparacaine hydrochloride ophthalmic eyedrops. Lead eye shields coated with an ophthalmic antibiotic ointment are then inserted beneath the eyelids.

Before large lesions are treated, a preliminary test patch area of approximately 1 cm^2 in a representative location is treated to confirm both the efficacy of the laser treatment and the patient's likelihood of scar formation. Although the predictive accuracy of a test patch area is not absolute, it is useful to the patient and the physician in assessing the results of laser surgery. The test patch treatment is performed approximately 12 weeks prior to regular treatment. Test patches are done in a 1 cm^2 area in a representative location to observe the amount of blanching and to determine whether scarring will occur. A test patch is not 100% predictive unless each separate anatomical area (cheek, lip, eyelid, scalp, etc.) is tested separately. The test patch also allows the patient to observe the course of healing and subsequent fading.

For definitive treatment, large lesions are divided into treatment segments of 2 to 3 in.^{2} corresponding to natural anatomic areas of the face. Treatment in segmental or intermittent patterns (such as "zebra striping," striping in broad bands, or point-by-point treatment) has not proved to reduce posttreatment complications substantially. In studies of large series of patients, the rate of complications (scars, hypopigmentation, texture changes, and so on) for those treated in an alternating pattern of rows and stripes was very similar to the rate for those patients treated in solid block areas. The possibility of a residual pattern of stripes and the unusual or bizarre appearance of the patient while undergoing treatment are also disadvantages of the stripe treatment method.

Immediate posttreatment care includes continuous application of ice compresses for six hours to enhance patient comfort and to minimize edema, exudate, and loss of capillary permeability. The patient is warned that there may be swelling of the treated areas, especially when laser surgery is performed in the periorbital area. Subsequent treatment may be similar to that following abrasion or superficial burn. The patient is advised to cleanse the wound daily with water and bacteriostatic liquid cleanser and to apply a topical antibiotic ointment. Systemic antibiotics are usually unnecessary. No makeup should be applied until the lesion has epithelialized.

The laser wound immediately after treatment appears as a gray-tan spot of blanched and coagulated blood vessels on the skin surface. Within several days, an eschar or scab forms that persists for seven to 14 days, during which epithelialization occurs. A period of laser burn erythema then follows, with some depression of the test spot; this stage persists variably for up to 12 weeks. At 12 weeks, slow progressive fading ensues that may continue for up to 12 months. Since delayed fading or blanching may occur as long as 12 months following treatment, no retreatment is indicated prior to this time. The patient is cautioned to avoid sun exposure and, once the crust is gone, to use total opaque sun block over the treated area to prevent the development of hyperpigmentation. The frequency and timing of postoperative visits will vary depending on such factors as the size of the lesion treated and the distance the patient lives from the physician. Generally, patients are seen at three-month and 12-month follow-up periods.

MECHANISM OF ACTION

The argon laser produces intense, bright blue-green light, which falls at 488 and 515 nm in the visible light spectrum. Because its frequency is considerably lower than that of x-ray or ultraviolet radiation, the argon laser is not expected to produce iatrogenic malignant neoplasms. For clinical use, a combination of blue (488 nm) and green (515 nm) light is used for more complete absorption. These wavelengths coincide with the maximum absorption curve of both hemoglobin and melanin, thus rendering argon laser light valuable in treating both cutaneous vascular and pigmented lesions (Fig 2–1).

The argon laser light has several unique properties that render it particularly valuable in the treatment of cutaneous lesions. It has the ability to penetrate the intact epidermis until it undergoes absorption by a pigmented structure in the dermis. This pigment can be hemoglobin, melanin, or the suspended pigment of tattoo or foreign-body particles. The laser light is converted to heat on absorption, and this heat produces a very selective coagulation or vaporization in the upper dermis. Adjacent dermal appendages (such as sweat glands and hair follicles) are relatively impervious to laser light and aid in the rapid healing and reepithelialization of the laser wound. The laser wound is initially similar to a superficial second-degree burn, with slough of the epidermis secondary to the heat produced in the subadjacent upper dermis. This burn is highly selective and is limited to the upper dermal layers, which ensures

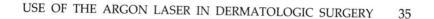

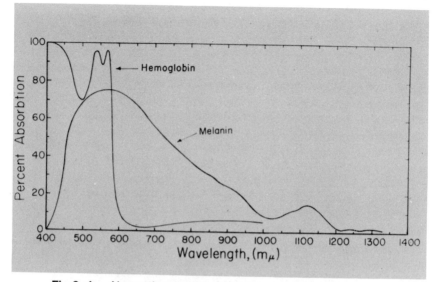

Fig 2–1.—Absorption spectrum for hemoglobin and melanin.

reepithelialization and healing of the wound from the dermal appendages.

Histopathologic sampling of laser wounds following treatment for hemangioma has shown that the large, ectatic vessels are obliterated in the upper 1 mm of the dermis. The dermal tissue has been replaced by a diffuse, collagenous deposit that contains only sparse, slitlike vessels that are frequently devoid of red blood cells. This layer is covered by a normal epidermis. These changes have been permanent and stable over an eight-year period of study (Figs 2–2 and 2–3).

The argon laser delivers appreciable energy only to the upper 1 mm of the dermis when used in the manner described in the previous section. Therefore, those port-wine hemangiomas that are confined to the upper dermis or above this layer respond favorably to the laser. Noe and associates reported on factors that predict the response of port-wine hemangioma to argon laser therapy, based on a study of 62 patients. Factors that favored a desirable result (marked lightening of the lesion without scarring) included the following: (1) patient's age greater than 37 years; (2) darker purple

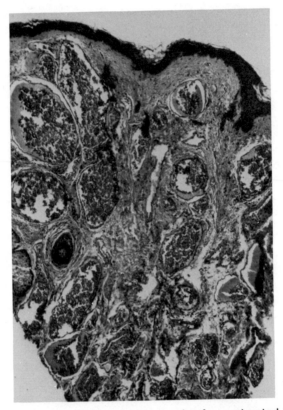

Fig 2–2.—Large ectatic dermal vessels of an untreated port-wine hemangioma.

color vs. pink (or lighter) color of port-wine hemangioma; (3) vascular area fraction of dermis occupied by vessels over 5%; (4) mean vessel area greater than 2,500 μm^2; and (5) percentage fullness (percentage of vessels containing erythrocytes) greater than 15%. Of all these factors, percentage fullness was determined to be the most critical and accurate. Based on these factors biopsy may be used to predict the success of laser therapy, but most experienced operators rely on clinical judgment to assess the expected results.

Electron microscopic examination immediately after laser impact shows collapse of the vascular lumina of the hemangioma, vacuolation and denaturation of both endothelial cells and karyocytes

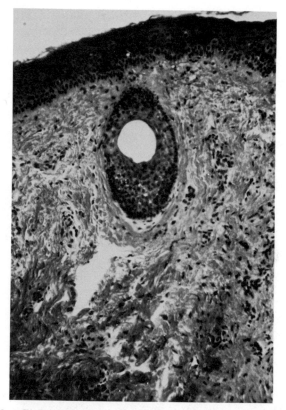

Fig 2–3.—Eight years following laser treatment of port-wine hemangioma, the epidermis is normal and the dermis contains a diffuse, collagenous deposit with few vessels.

(as well as fibrocytes and other cells in the upper dermis), and apparent fractionation of the vascular basal membranes. With healing, the residual vessels have abnormally thick, collagenous walls and very poorly defined basement membranes with permanent endothelial cell damage but otherwise lack distinctive features.

The laser is equally effective in the treatment of decorative or traumatic tattoos. Tattoo pigment selectively absorbs laser light regardless of pigment color or composition. The pigment then vaporizes as a laser plume, rather than producing the photocoagulatory effect seen in hemangioma treatment. This vaporization of foreign-body pigment is then followed by a macrophage phagocytic inflammatory phase. Once again, the absorption of the laser light is selective and is restricted to dermal pigment, sparing epidermis and dermal appendages. Histopathologic sampling of laser wounds after treatment of tattoos has shown that the pigment is obliterated in the upper 1 mm of the dermis, and is replaced by a diffuse, collagenous deposit covered by a normal epidermis (Figs 2–4 and 2–5).

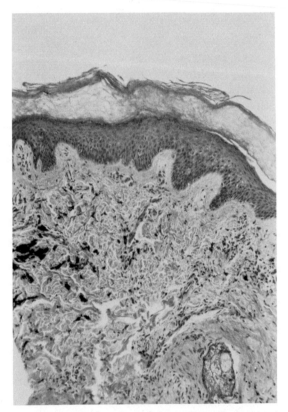

Fig 2–4.—Untreated tattoo, demonstrating pigment suspended in upper dermis.

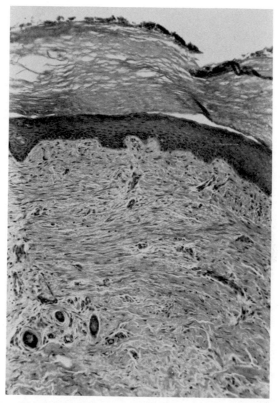

Fig 2–5.—Treated tattoo, with collagen in upper dermis and loss of tattoo pigment.

REVIEW OF PATIENT DATA

Table 2–1 shows the categories of lesions that have proved amenable to argon laser treatment and gives treatment parameters and results. Major categories include superficial vascular lesions, decorative tattoos, inflammatory lesions, and miscellaneous benign skin lesions.

TABLE 2-1.—CLINICAL LASER SUMMARY

LESION	NO. OF PATIENTS	SPOT SIZE (MM)	AVERAGE NO. OF TREATMENTS	PULSE DURATION (SEC)	POWER (WATTS)	RESULTS (%)		
						GOOD	POOR	SCAR
Vascular lesions								
Port-wine hemangioma	1,400	1.0–5.0	4.8	0.2–20.0	0.5–1.5	75	25	14
Capillary/cavernous hemangioma	105	1.0–5.0	1.4	2.0–6.0	1.0–2.0	86	14	5
Telangiectasia (face)	370	0.2–1.0	1.2	1.0–2.0	0.8–1.2	99	1	0
Acne rosacea	18	1.0–5.0	3.0	2.0–10.0	1.0–1.5	90	10	0
Campbell De Morgan senile angioma	12	0.2–2.0	2.0	2.0–8.0	1.0–1.5	100	0	0
Venous lakes	9	1.0–2.0	1.0	1.0–6.0	1.0–1.5	100	0	0
Strawberry hemangioma	8	1.0–5.0	2.0	5.0–20.0	1.5–2.0	70	30	35
Tattoo								
Decorative	190	0.2–2.0	3.8	20.0	1.0–2.5	53	47	34
Traumatic	3	1.0–2.0	1.0	2.0–4.0	1.5	100	0	0
Inflammatory lesions								
Pyogenic granuloma	7	1.0–2.0	1.0	5.0–20.0	1.5–2.3	100	0	0
Granuloma faciale	3	1.0–2.0	4.3	4.0–10.0	1.0–1.8	75	25	0
Miscellaneous								
Nevi of Ota	9	1.0–2.0	3.7	4.0–8.0	0.8–1.4	60	40	0
Hereditary hemorrhagic telangiectasia	8	1.0	4.3	1.0–3.0	1.0	95	5	0
Angio ford	1	1.0	2.0	1.0–2.0	1.0	100	0	0
Trichoepithelioma	1	1.0–2.0	3.0	6.0–10.0	1.2–1.8	100	0	0

Vascular Lesions

The treatment of cutaneous vascular lesions, especially port-wine hemangiomas, was the primary purpose for, and remains the mainstay of, the argon laser treatment program. The majority of port-wine hemangiomas appear on the face, but these congenital vascular lesions can also occur on the trunk, neck, and upper and lower extremities. Syndromes associated with port-wine hemangiomas (such as Sturge-Weber syndrome) are present in approximately 5% of patients.

An intensive pretreatment consultation visit is carried out with the patient and family. At this time, the procedure, reasonable expectations, and the possibility of scarring are discussed in detail. It should be emphasized that while the argon laser will result in a lightening of the port-wine hemangioma, the treated area will not be normal-appearing skin. An individual treatment sheet is started for each patient and the patient is given a written explanation of the condition and proposed treatment method to take home. These forms are reproduced in Appendices A, B, and C. Photographs are taken of all lesions preoperatively and at follow-up visits. A Kodak color bar included in the photograph is helpful to use as a color reference in comparing photographs of different exposures.

Laser treatment of port-wine hemangiomas of the face, scalp, and neck results in marked blanching and lightening without scars in approximately 70% of treated patients (Figs 2–6 and 2–7). An eschar forms immediately postoperatively and lasts seven to 14 days. The treated area first appears pale and depressed, then may turn red. Over the next three to 12 months, the treated area will progressively lighten. In addition, the deforming hypertrophy that many of these lesions undergo in later life may be markedly reduced with laser surgery (Figs 2–8 and 2–9). Similar lesions of the trunk and extremities are less responsive to argon laser treatment and result in very modest lightening and a higher incidence of scarring; for this reason, they are usually excluded from treatment. Port-wine stains in patients under age 12 to 15 years also fade only modestly with a higher incidence of scarring and are thus excluded from treatment. The argon laser has the ability to enhance or improve previously unsuccessful treatment (e.g., reverse dermal tattooing) or to be adjunctive to previous partial or incomplete treatment (e.g.,

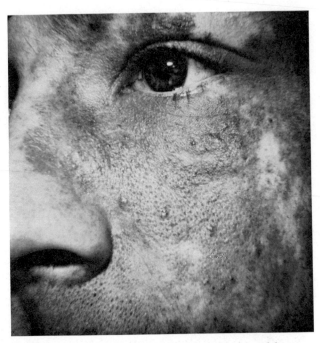

Fig 2–6.—Port-wine hemangioma of side of face.

incomplete resection with flap or graft resurfacing). Complications of argon laser treatment of port-wine hemangiomas include hypopigmentation (occurring in 28% of patients), skin texture changes (22%), and hypertrophic scarring, particularly in the perioral and nasolabial areas (15%) (Figs 2–10 and 2–11).

Other cutaneous vascular abnormalities that are amenable to argon laser treatment include superficial capillary/cavernous hemangiomas, telangiectasias, and Campbell De Morgan senile angiomas (Figs 2–12 to 2–15). The rosacea (telangiectatic) component of acne rosacea can be easily blanched by the laser; but the thick, oily, irregular skin (the acneiform component, or rhinophyma) is not changed by argon laser treatment (Figs 2–16 and 2–17). Capillary hemangiomas of infancy ("strawberry marks") have been treated for indications of bleeding, ulceration, or infection or for obstruction of

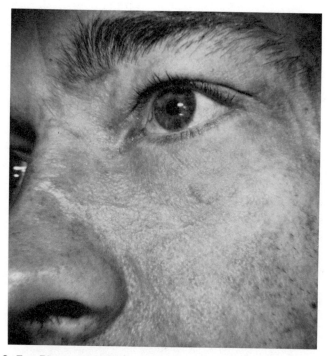

Fig 2–7.—Photocoagulation and blanching of hemangioma following laser treatment (same patient as in Fig 2–6).

a vital bodily orifice (Figs 2–18 and 2–19). Telangiectasias of the nose and nasolabial folds treated with the argon laser may heal with grooving or indentation at the hyperpigmented sites of the telangiectasias.

Telangiectasias or superficial varicosities of the lower extremities are not responsive to laser treatment. The treated areas appear purple and depressed, often leaving a worse cosmetic appearance than the untreated condition.

The argon laser has been used successfully to treat the postrhinoplasty "red nose syndrome." The clinical picture is one of diffuse redness of the nose, with multiple minute ectatic vessels. The vessels are so small that the entire areas must be treated rather than individual vessels.

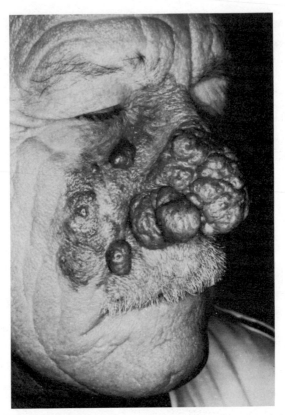

Fig 2–8.—Marked hypertrophy and deformity associated with long-standing port-wine hemangioma.

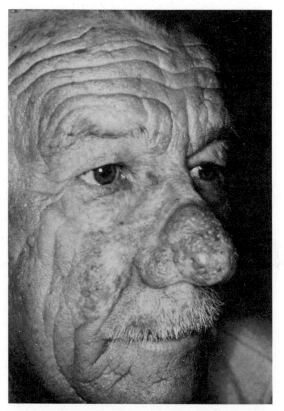

Fig 2–9.—Marked smoothening and restoration of contour following laser treatment of port-wine hemangioma (same patient as in Fig 2–8).

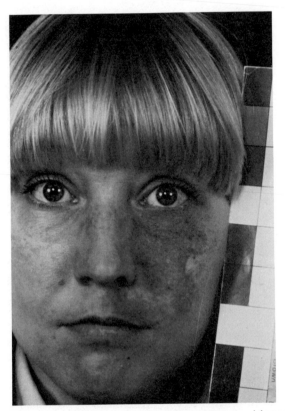

Fig 2–10.—Port-wine hemangioma in a 22-year-old woman.

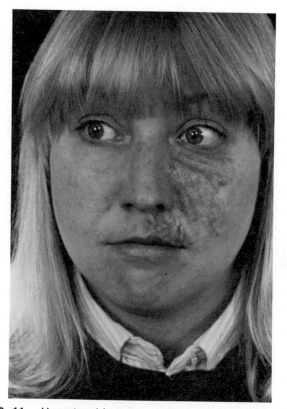

Fig 2–11.—Hypertrophic scar on cheek and upper lip following treatment of port-wine hemangioma (same patient as in Fig 2–10).

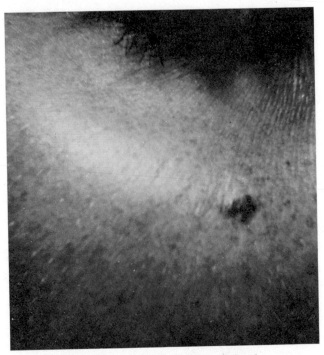

Fig 2–12.—Telangiectasia on cheek.

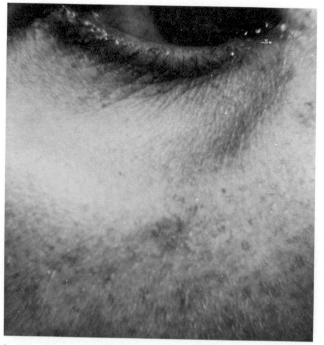

Fig 2–13.—Total obliteration of telangiectasia without recurrence or scar (same patient as in Fig 2–12).

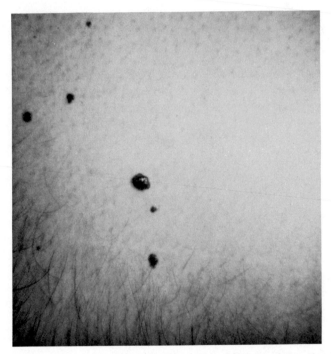

Fig 2–14.—Campbell De Morgan senile angioma of the chest.

Fig 2–15.—Blanching of angiomas without recurrence or scar (same patient as in Fig 2–14).

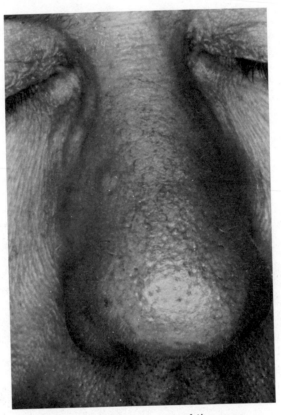

Fig 2–16.—Acne rosacea of the nose.

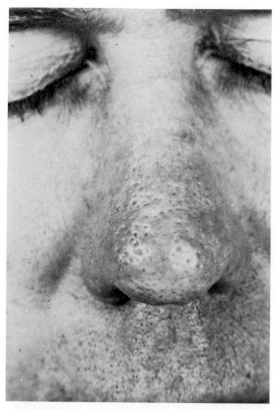

Fig 2–17.—Satisfactory obliteration of red blood vessels after laser treatment of acne rosacea with no change in sebaceous skin (same patient as in Fig 2–16).

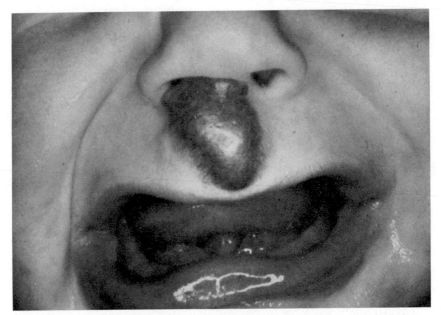

Fig 2–18.—"Strawberry mark" (capillary hemangioma of infancy) on philtrum of 2-year-old child prior to treatment.

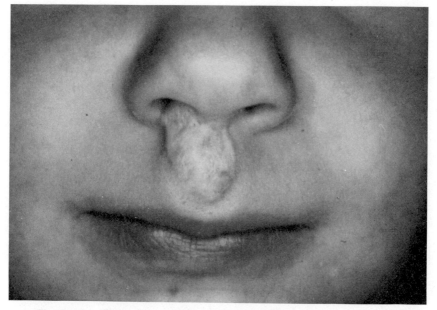

Fig 2–19.—Flattening and blanching of lesion (same patient as in Fig 2–18) following laser treatment of "strawberry mark."

Decorative Tattoo

Argon laser treatment of decorative tattoos is a simple, efficient outpatient procedure using local anesthesia. The results are comparable to or minimally superior to other, conventional methods, which may be more time consuming or more complicated, requiring multiple stages, graft or flap coverage, or general anesthesia (Figs 2–20 and 2–21). Shortcomings of argon laser treatment of tattoos include permanent changes in skin texture (100% of patients), residual "ghost" tattoo pigmentation in small areas (50%), and hypertrophic scarring. Hypertrophic scarring may be present in over 30% of patients seen at three months but dramatically resolves with pressure, time, and steroid injections to approximately 20% in 12 months. To place these figures in perspective, one should recall that the majority of tattoo treatments are performed in areas of traditionally difficult wound healing with resultant hypertrophic scarring,

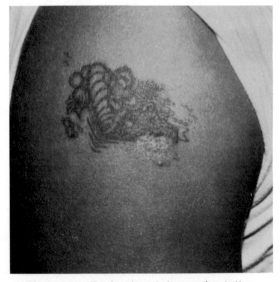

Fig 2–20.—Professional decorative tattoo.

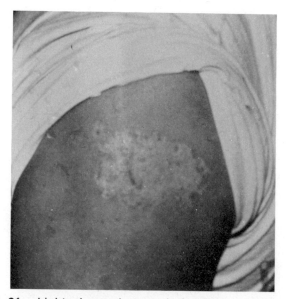

Fig 2–21.—Lightening and removal of majority of tattoo pigment (same tattoo as shown in Fig 2–20) with residual skin texture change.

such as the deltoid and forearm area of the arm, the hand, the back and trunk, and the lower extremities.

Inflammatory Lesions

Inflammatory lesions usually consist of nests and masses of capillaries in an edematous matrix in the subepidermal or superficial dermal area. This abnormal collection of hemoglobin-laden vessels and inflammatory cells under the skin attracts and absorbs blue-green laser light much as the ectatic vessels in port-wine hemangiomas do. Thus, heat coagulation and subsequent involution of the inflammatory component results. Pyogenic granulomas are uniquely amenable to laser treatment, as the superficial granulation-like character of the dense inflammatory vessels attracts the laser (Figs 2–22 and 2–23). Other inflammatory lesions, such as granuloma faciale, are also responsive to the argon laser.

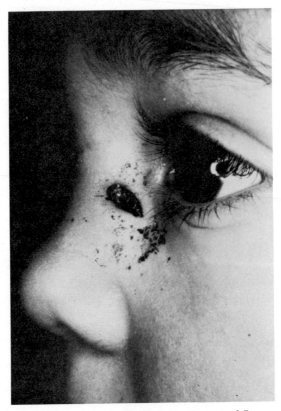

Fig 2–22.—Pyogenic granuloma on side of nose of 5-year-old child.

Miscellaneous Benign Lesions

An ever-widening variety of benign cutaneous lesions is amenable to argon laser treatment. Oculodermal melanosis (nevus of Ota) can be partially lightened by the laser. Numerous patients with hereditary hemorrhagic telangiectasia (Rendu-Osler-Weber disease) have had superficial cutaneous or oral membrane telangiectasias cleared by laser light. Oral (lip, tongue, or palate) telangiectasias that may bleed with tooth brushing or rough diet can be eradicated by such treatment. In addition, nasal mucosal lesions that cause recurrent and occasionally severe epistaxis can be improved by laser

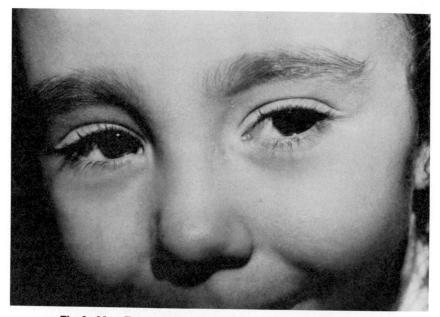

Fig 2–23.—Total obliteration of pyogenic granuloma, without recurrence or scarring (same patient as in Fig 2–22).

treatment. The argon laser does not completely eliminate any further bleeding; it merely decreases the amount and severity of the epistaxis. Patients report fewer nosebleeds, more frequent hemorrhage-free intervals, greatly decreased heavy bleeding during occasional nosebleeds, and greater ease and speed in stopping bleeding. It should be emphasized that hereditary hemorrhagic telangiectasia is a relentlessly progressive disease, and argon laser treatment is not a permanent cure but merely a palliative procedure to decrease the frequency and severity of the bleeding. Repeated laser treatments may be necessary at three- to six-month intervals.

Miscellaneous lesions such as facial trichoepithelioma (Figs 2–24 and 2–25), scrotal angiokeratomas, and adenoma sebaceum can also be successfully treated by the laser. Trichoepithelioma, which is colorless, takes advantage of the vaporization effect of continuous, long-duration laser exposure rather than the color-specific absorption by hemoglobin or melanin.

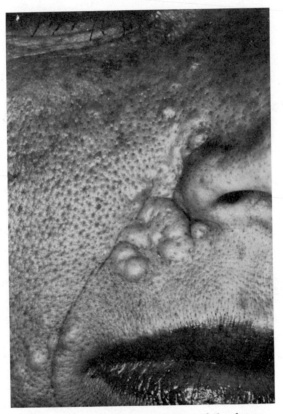

Fig 2–24.—Trichoepithelioma of the face.

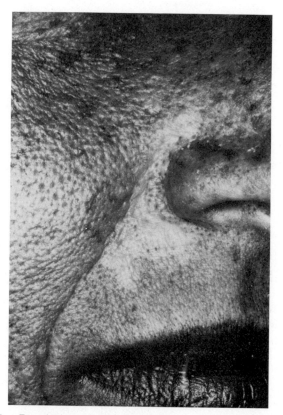

Fig 2–25.—Resolution of trichoepithelioma of the face 12 months after treatment (same patient as in Fig 2–24).

SUMMARY

The argon laser has found a definite place in the armamentarium of the dermatologist or plastic surgeon in the treatment of a wide variety of benign cutaneous lesions. In some cases (e.g., telangiectasia, tattoo) the laser is equivalent to the more standard current methods of treatment, and in other cases (e.g., acne rosacea, hereditary hemorrhagic telangiectasia) it is definitely a superior modality. Occasionally (e.g., for port-wine hemangiomas, trichoepithelioma, granuloma faciale, and nevus of Ota), the laser has proved to be the only effective treatment modality when all others have been insufficient or ineffectual. As time and experience progress, the laser will undoubtedly assume a commonplace role in the mainstream treatment of a variety of cutaneous or superficial lesions and will become the method of choice for many such lesions.

BIBLIOGRAPHY

Apfelberg, D. B., et al. Analysis of complications of argon laser treatment for port wine hemangiomas with reference to striped technique. *Lasers Surg. Med.* 2:357–371, 1983.

Apfelberg, D. B., et al. Expanded role of the argon laser in plastic surgery. *J. Dermatol. Surg. Oncol.* 9:145–151, 1983.

Apfelberg, D. B., et al. Granuloma faciale—treatment with argon laser. *Arch. Dermatol.* 119:573–576, 1983.

Apfelberg, D. B., et al. Histology of port wine stains following argon laser treatment. *Br. J. Plast. Surg.* 32:232–237, 1979.

Apfelberg, D. B., et al. Pathophysiology and treatment of decorative tattoos with reference to argon laser treatment. *Clin. Plast. Surg.* 7:369–377, 1980.

Apfelberg, D., et al. Progress report on extended clinical use of the argon laser for cutaneous lesions. *Lasers Surg. Med.* 1:71, 1980.

Apfelberg, D. B., et al. Results of argon laser exposure of capillary hemangiomas of infancy—preliminary report. *Plast. Reconstr. Surg.* 67:188–193, 1981.

Apfelberg, D. B., et al. Study of carcinogenic effects of in vitro argon laser exposure of fibroblasts. *Plast. Reconstr. Surg.* 71:93–97, 1983.

Apfelberg, D. B., et al. The argon laser for cutaneous lesions. *J.A.M.A.* 245:2073–2075, 1981.

Apfelberg, D. B., et al. Update on laser usage in treatment of decorative tattoos. *Lasers Surg. Med.* 2:169–177, 1983.

Apfelberg, D. B.; Maser, M. R.; and Lash, H. Argon laser management of cutaneous vascular deformities—a preliminary report. *West. J. Med.* 124:99–101, 1981.

Apfelberg, D. B.; Maser, M. R.; and Lash, H. Argon laser treatment of decorative tattoos. *Br. J. Plast. Surg.* 32:141–144, 1979.

Apfelberg, D. B.; Maser, M. R.; and Lash, H. Extended clinical use of the argon laser for cutaneous lesions. *Arch. Dermatol.* 115:719–721, 1979.

Arndt, K. A. Argon laser therapy of small cutaneous vascular lesions. *Arch. Dermatol.* 118:220–224, 1982.

Cosman, B. Clinical experience in the laser therapy of port wine stains. *Lasers Surg. Med.* 1:133–152, 1980.

Cosman, B. Experience in the argon laser therapy of port wine stains. *Plast. Reconstr. Surg.* 65:119–129, 1980.

Gilchrist, B. A.; Rosen, S.; and Noe, J. M. Chilling port wine stains improves the response to argon laser therapy. *Plast. Reconstr. Surg.* 69:278–283, 1982.

Goldman, L., et al. Treatment of port wine marks by an argon laser. *J. Dermatol. Surg. Oncol.* 2:385–388, 1976.

McBurney, E. I., and Leonard, G. I. Argon laser treatment of port-wine hemangiomas: clinical and histologic correlation. *South. Med. J.* 74:925–927, 1981.

Noe, J. M., et al. Port wine stains and the response to argon laser therapy: successful treatment and the predictive role of color, age, and biopsy. *Plast. Reconstr. Surg.* 65:130–136, 1980.

Noe, J. M., et al. Post rhinoplasty "red nose": differential diagnosis and treatment by laser. *Plast. Reconstr. Surg.* 67:661–664, 1981.

APPENDIX A

INDIVIDUAL TREATMENT SHEET

Argon Laser Photocoagulation

PATIENT _____ DATE _____

DIAGNOSIS _____ TREATMENT BY _____

SKIN PIGMENT _____ DATA BY _____

INITIAL DATE OF INQUIRY _____

Age lesion first appeared _____

Changes in lesion _____

Previous treatments _____

Associated medical problems _____

Drug allergies _____

Family history _____

Exact size, color, extent of lesion _____

Makeup _____

Referred by _____

DATE	BIOPSY	AREA TREATED (size)	PHOTO	SPOT SIZE (mm)	EXPOSURE TIME (sec)	POWER (watts)	NO. OF EXPOSURES	MISCELLANEOUS

65

APPENDIX B

WHAT IS A PORT-WINE HEMANGIOMA?

A port-wine hemangioma is an abnormal collection or network of blood vessels present beneath a layer of otherwise normal skin. This dense network of vessels is a remainder of extra blood vessel tissue that was present during the first month of embryologic life. The port-wine hemangioma was so named because the skin appears as though a red, pink, or purple liquid, such as port wine, had been poured over it.

WHAT IS THE NATURAL HISTORY OF A PORT-WINE HEMANGIOMA?

Port-wine hemangiomas are present on the skin at birth and appear to grow at the same rate as the surrounding tissues. In other words, they keep pace with the normal adjacent skin as far as size is concerned, but in the third, fourth, or fifth decades of life they may become thicker or spongier than the adjacent normal skin. Furthermore, the surface of the hemangioma, which may have been quite smooth during the first decades of life, may develop an irregular and lumpy "cobblestone street" appearance by the time the patient is in his 40s, 50s, or 60s. Fortunately, these hemangiomas are neither dangerous nor malignant.

WHAT TREATMENTS ARE AVAILABLE FOR PORT-WINE HEMANGIOMAS?

Many forms of therapy have been used on port-wine hemangiomas in the past; most have been abandoned, either because they are ineffective or because they create another deformity that is as undesirable as the port-wine hemangioma itself. Surgeons have removed these areas and then reconstructed the defect with flaps or skin grafts. Such procedures entail a substantial amount of surgery, and the scars that result are often quite objectionable. X-rays, used in the past, are known to be potentially dangerous and are no longer used to treat port-wine hemangiomas. A variety of agents have been injected into the involved skin, but without any considerable success. Also ineffective has been the use of dry ice and carbon dioxide. Tattooing has been tried to camouflage these hemangiomas, but this method of treatment appears to be temporary and merely camouflages the birthmark.

HOW DOES THE ARGON LASER WORK?

The argon laser generates a very powerful light that is blue-green in color. It carries enormous energy that may be finely focused. When this light contacts the skin, the red color of the birthmark absorbs the light, which then releases its energy as heat. The heat coagulates, or cauterizes, the small vessels under the skin. In theory, the overlying skin is not affected by the laser. As a practical matter, however, the intense heat produced by the reaction to the laser light often causes a burnlike reaction in the skin, which must then heal.

WHAT IS THE SEQUENCE OF HEALING AFTER A LASER TREATMENT?

An immediate effect of the laser treatment is that tiny blood vessels under the skin are coagulated, causing the area to turn a much lighter color. Within a few days, a scab or crust will form, and this crust usually persists for approximately two weeks. During this two-week time, the patient should apply antibiotic ointment as directed by the physician and should attempt to keep the area as clean and dry as possible, avoiding strenuous physical activity that would cause excessive sweating. The crust or scab should be allowed to stay in place until it separates spontaneously; the patient should not pick at the scab. After the scab has separated, the area may be light in color; within several weeks, however, this treated area will again become red. It may appear at this time as if the hemangioma has recurred, but such is not the case. Rather, it is the usual reaction of the skin to the laser light exposure. The redness then gradually fades over the next several months. At that point, when the redness has faded, the full effect of the laser treatment is usually readily seen. There may be a slight depression in the skin of the treated area. This depression usually becomes smoother as healing progresses.

WHAT ARE THE HAZARDS, COMPLICATIONS, AND LIMITATIONS OF ARGON LASER TREATMENT?

There are several potential hazards and limitations in this treatment program. It is important to realize that the argon laser does not completely eliminate a hemangioma. There is no way the argon laser can totally erase a birthmark that has been on the skin for many years. At best, the laser may cause a marked lightening of the birthmark, so that birthmarks that are deep purple may become light violet, and birthmarks that are deep red will often become light pink. Usually, patients are able to switch from a thick, heavy makeup, such as Covermark, to one that is more normal and easier to apply. In no case has the laser been able to eliminate the birthmark totally. The laser appears to improve the sponginess and irregularities of the skin that appear over the years. This effect, however, is not certain, as it may take 20 to 30 years of follow-up of laser-treated patients before we are able to determine the accuracy of this finding.

Another potential limitation of the laser treatment is that a number of patients have had some scarring, such as may occur with a burn. The scar may appear raised, red, or white. The scarring may fade somewhat with time but may never completely disappear.

Finally, there is no way of predicting what long-term, undesirable, or unusual side effects may occur as a result of laser light treatments. Every new treatment method raises the possibility that unsuspected side effects may be created that will not become evident for many years following the treatment. One should realize, however, that many types of lasers have been used in medicine for over 15 years, and thus far there is no evidence of unsuspected side effects; this finding does not guarantee that they will not occur or be discovered at some time in the distant future.

COSTS OF TREATMENT AND INSURANCE COVERAGE

There is no guarantee that medical insurance will cover the costs of laser treatments. Some insurance companies may consider the treatment purely cosmetic. Each patient or patient's family should check with the insurance carrier to determine whether treatments will be covered. A letter from the physician explaining that the treatment is reconstructive rather than cosmetic may be helpful in obtaining benefits from the insurance carrier. Treatment fees will be discussed with each patient at the time of consultation, and questions regarding such fees are welcome.

APPENDIX C

LASER TREATMENT CARE INSTRUCTIONS

1. Expect a crust or scab to appear over the treatment area 24 to 72 hours after laser treatment and to last approximately 7 to 14 days.
2. Keep the area clean and dry until the crust or scab comes off.
3. Do not pick the crust or scab.
4. While the crust or scab is present, very sparingly apply the prescribed antibiotic ointment. This treatment can be discontinued after all crusts or scabs come off. Makeup can be applied after the scab comes off.
5. Avoid bright sunlight to the area by the use of sunscreen agents containing PABA or by wearing hats with brims or visors for at least six months.
6. After the scab or crust comes off, the area may appear pale and depressed or indented. The area may then turn red after several weeks and may stay depressed or indented. This redness usually gradually fades in one year.
7. Keep us informed about the progress of the treated area by a letter and photograph six weeks from your treatment date. It is also especially important for us to receive a letter and photograph two weeks before your return visit. *No follow-up appointments can be made without this correspondence.* (In the past, some patients have traveled to our facility only to find that the treated area was not well enough healed to allow further treatments. This unnecessary time and expense can be avoided by correspondence prior to the follow-up visit.)

71

3

USE OF THE CARBON DIOXIDE LASER IN DERMATOLOGIC SURGERY

PHILIP L. BAILIN, M.D.

JOHN LOUIS RATZ, M.D.

THE CARBON dioxide (CO_2) laser is truly a remarkably versatile instrument when applied to the field of dermatologic surgery. It may serve as a "light scalpel" for accomplishing incisional or excisional procedures. It may also be used for the superficial vaporization of the skin surface, removing only a thin layer of cells with each pass of beam. What is most remarkable is that the operator may accomplish these two entirely different applications by merely moving the surgical handpiece closer to or farther from the cutaneous surface.

The techniques and applications of the two modes of therapy with the CO_2 laser are explained in detail in subsequent sections of this chapter. But first, a brief review of the structure and mechanism of action of the CO_2 laser is in order.

MECHANISM OF ACTION

The CO_2 laser is a gas laser that uses a mixture of carbon dioxide, nitrogen, and helium as the lasing medium. The light output from all of the commercially available units is of a continuous type; no pulsed or switched formats currently exist. Excitation of the lasing medium is most commonly achieved by a high-voltage electrical charge. Recently, however, new technology has enabled certain manufacturers to achieve excitation by means of a radio frequency wave. This technique has engendered the production of smaller units that do not require the continuous addition of a fresh supply of carbon dioxide gas mixture. This technology has been especially helpful in allowing the design of units small and mobile enough to function easily in the dermatologist's office.

A feature common to all of the dermatologic CO_2 laser systems is the delivery of the laser light beam to the tissue through an articulated arm device that contains a series of reflecting mirrors (Fig 3–1). No optical fiber system currently is available that can efficiently and safely carry light of the CO_2 laser wavelength, at 10,600

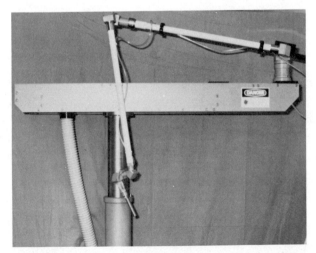

Fig 3–1.—Articulated arm extends from the end of the plasma tube and contains a system of reflecting mirrors. This device is typical of most CO_2 lasers used in cutaneous surgery.

nm. The articulated arm configuration terminates in the reasonably small and lightweight surgical handpiece, which is usually arranged on a multiple joint to allow several degrees of freedom of rotation for the operator (Fig 3–2). The beam exits this handpiece through a lens with a given focal length. The lens may be changeable, or the entire handpiece/lens unit may be changeable. The focal length is important, as it determines the working distance from the skin surface for various applications, as will be explained later.

The light beam output of the CO_2 laser is invisible to the naked eye, as it lies in the far-infrared portion of the electromagnetic spectrum. This very basic fact proved to be quite a problem for the early users of the CO_2 laser, since they had to estimate where the beam would strike the skin and whether it was in exact focus or defocused. All the recent commercially available units have overcome this serious problem by incorporating a coaxial aiming beam. This aiming beam is most commonly a red beam produced by a very low power helium-neon laser incorporated into the instrument. The addition of this beam makes aiming and focusing (or defocusing) the

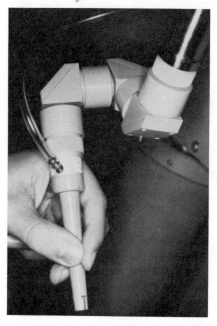

Fig 3–2.—Articulated arm ends in the surgical handpiece, which is usually mounted on a multiple joint for freedom of rotation.

CO_2 beam quite a simple matter. The helium-neon beam has absolutely no biologic effects.

The action of the CO_2 laser light beam on tissue requires some explanation. Since this beam of light is colorless (far-infrared), there is no selective absorption of the light by various colors in the target tissue. Rather, the light is uniformly absorbed. It is also important to note that this wavelength of light is absorbed even by a transparent medium, such as water. This characteristic of the CO_2 laser is in marked contrast to the action of the argon laser beam or the Nd-YAG beam, which are transmitted through clear mediums without much absorption.

The skin is approximately 90% water in content. As the beam strikes the skin, the intracellular and extracellular water absorb the energy of the light in an instantaneous fashion. This absorption results in the immediate conversion of the water to tissue steam, which causes the tissue to vaporize instantly. The rapidity of this phenomenon precludes the transfer of any substantial amount of heat energy to the adjacent tissue. For this reason, the tissue receiving the impact of the laser beam is totally destroyed, while the cells immediately next to or beneath the site of impact are essentially undamaged. This process naturally results in the most precise and localized form of tissue ablation.

The beam of the CO_2 laser has two other physical characteristics that enhance its precision as an ablative tool. First, the beam exhibits virtually no internal scatter within tissue. By contrast, the argon laser beam exhibits about 100 times the amount of scatter. Second, the CO_2 laser beam has a coefficient of extinction in tissue of approximately 0.1 mm. (By comparison, the coefficient of extinction for the argon laser is 2 to 3 mm.) This measurement refers to the depth in a given medium (e.g., water or tissue) at which a laser beam passing through is totally absorbed. Beyond this depth there is no further beam transmission and consequently no further beam effect. The smaller the coefficient of extinction, the more superficial and focal the laser's effect will be.

In addition to its remarkable precision, the CO_2 laser has other features that make it a most desirable surgical instrument. As the beam incises or vaporizes tissue, it seals blood vessels. The caliber of the vessels spontaneously sealed by this beam has been estimated at a maximum diameter of 0.5 to 1.5 mm. This spontaneous sealing produces relatively hemostatic surgery in most cases. Darker vessels that are severed may be grasped by a forceps, and their ends may be sealed with the laser beam defocused to an impact spot of 1 to 2 mm. It is thought that lymphatic vessels may be sealed in a similar fashion.

The beam is also known to sterilize the surgical field as it cuts. Furthermore, the cutaneous nerves that are transected by the beam as it is cutting behave differently than those cut by cold steel or by an electrosurgical tool. The cut ends seen ultrastructurally after the latter injury appear to be "frayed." Those ends seen after laser injury appear to be capped or welded over. This difference is thought to account for the markedly decreased level of pain after most CO_2 laser surgical procedures.

While there are obviously many advantages to using the CO_2 laser for skin surgery, there are also potential disadvantages. The one that has caused the greatest concern relates to wound strength after surgery. Recent studies have demonstrated, however, that wounds produced by the CO_2 laser achieve the same tensile strength as cold steel wounds by 21 days. Thus, the relative weakness of the laser wound is only temporary. This concern seems to be more theoretical than practical, as there are almost no documented cases of wound dehiscence after CO_2 laser surgery.

Now that the mechanism of action of the CO_2 laser has been discussed, we turn to a consideration of the use of this instrument as an incisional, or cutting, tool.

EXCISION

For all incisional applications of the CO_2 laser it is necessary to work in the focused mode. For any given surgical handpiece/lens unit there is a fixed focal length. This focal length tells the operator the exact distance from the target tissue surface at which the laser handpiece must be held (or the internal lens must be located) to achieve precise focus on that surface (Fig 3–3). In addition, each system normally denotes the exact diameter of the laser beam at the impact spot on the tissue surface when it is in perfect focus. Most CO_2 laser systems currently in use for dermatologic surgery employ an impact spot at focality of 0.1 to 0.2 mm. Larger focal impact spots

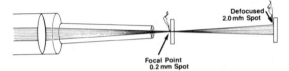

Fig 3–3.—A lens with characteristic focal length sits in the CO_2 laser handpiece, causing the once-parallel beam of light to converge to its focal point and then to diverge. Spot sizes shown are typical. The 0.2-mm spot at focality is for excisional use, while the 2.0-mm defocused spot is commonly used for vaporization.

are available with different lens systems, but these sizes are essentially too large for incisional purposes.

The handpiece/lens system need not be changed to allow the operator to go from focused beam incisional work to unfocused beam vaporizational work. All that is required is to move the handpiece either closer to or farther from the skin surface to defocus the beam. This change in distance produces two simultaneous effects. First, the diameter of the beam at the tissue impact site enlarges. Second, the power density of the beam decreases. This decrease occurs, of course, because the same beam power is now falling on a larger area of tissue than at the focal point (Fig 3–4).

The simple physical facts described in the preceding paragraphs endow the CO_2 laser system with amazing versatility and ease of operation. By merely moving the handpiece toward and away from the skin, without any changes of power at the console, the operator can vary the tissue effects and can go back and forth from incision to vaporization.

We may now proceed to the actual incisional applications of the CO_2 laser. All such procedures may be performed in a standard outpatient surgical treatment room, provided the basic laser safety measures have been taken. These measures include appropriate signs on the door of the room, an interruption prevention system (usually a simple internal door lock), and proper eye protection for all in the room. There must also be adequate provision for smoke evacuation, since the CO_2 laser produces a constant plume of smoke as it destroys tissue. This evacuation may be accomplished by a built-in suction vacuum system, as is found in hospital operating suites; more commonly for dermatologic applications, however, a small, portable laser smoke evacuation unit is used. These units are

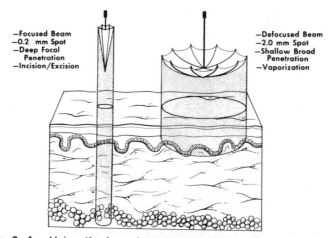

-Focused Beam
-0.2 mm Spot
-Deep Focal
  Penetration
-Incision/Excision

-Defocused Beam
-2.0 mm Spot
-Shallow Broad
  Penetration
-Vaporization

Fig 3-4.—Using the laser beam at the focal point concentrates the energy into a small area with relatively deep penetration, analogous to dropping a closed umbrella onto a soft target. Drawing the handpiece back from the target defocuses the beam, spreading out the energy delivered. The impact site is larger but quite shallow. This mode is analogous to dropping an opened umbrella onto a soft target.

commercially available from several sources and function like vacuum cleaners. They usually contain activated charcoal filters as well as moisture absorbing filters.

The operative site may be prepared preoperatively as for standard surgery. All procedures are performed under local anesthesia, but the inclusion of vasoconstrictor substances such as epinephrine is not necessary, owing to the hemostatic cutting capability of the CO_2 laser. For additional safety, the skin surfaces adjacent to the immediate surgical field may be covered with drapes or gauzes lightly moistened in water or saline (Fig 3-5). These drapes act as a barrier to the beam should it accidentally be aimed away from the appropriate target. Draping is especially important in areas of the face consisting of irregularly contoured surfaces, such that the beam may easily overshoot one tissue plane and strike another (for example, a beam aimed at the edge of the nasal bridge may strike the adjacent cheek). A further caution would be the use of nonreflective instruments such as forceps, to avoid the potential reflection of the beam away from the operative field.

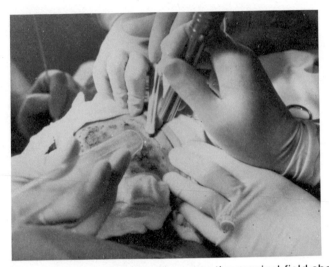

Fig 3–5.—Skin immediately adjacent to the surgical field should be covered with moistened dressings to protect the underlying tissue from accidental injury by the laser.

The choice of the CO_2 laser for incisional work could theoretically be universal. In truth, though, the size of the equipment and the need for additional personnel and equipment will probably limit its use to certain specific situations in which it offers a considerable advantage over cold steel or electrosurgical apparatus. The most common situation of this type is the excision of lesions in which bleeding would likely be a problem. The problem could be due to the patient's own physical condition, as in hypertension, anticoagulant therapy, a bleeding disorder, or a cardiac pacemaker precluding the use of a coagulator. It might be due to the nature of the lesion being excised, as in angioma, angiosarcoma, or large friable cutaneous carcinoma. It might also be a factor of the anatomic site, as in surgery of the scalp, lateral neck, temporal region, nose, or penis. In all such cases, the CO_2 laser gives a reliable degree of hemostasis as it cuts without substantial thermal necrosis of the tissue bed.

To achieve an incision that is fine and clean, resembling that produced by cold steel, takes considerable practice. The beam must be precisely focused to a fine spot of 0.1 to 0.2 mm in diameter, and, most important, it must be kept at precise focus throughout the

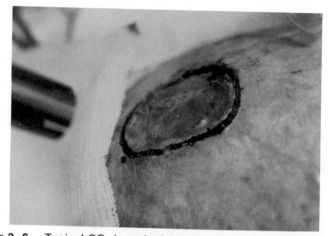

Fig 3–6.—Typical CO_2 laser incision is usually hemostatic. The laser should be held in focus throughout the incisional procedure.

length of the cut (Fig 3–6). If the operator allows his or her hand to wander in and out from the surface while moving the beam along the incision line, the laser will not give a pure cut. Rather, a mixture of cutting and vaporizing will occur, which results in an uneven incision line in terms of depth and width. The speed of the cut is also critical. Assuming that the beam is maintained in proper focus at all times, the speed of cutting (moving along the surface) is inversely proportional to the depth of the cut and the degree of hemostasis. In other words, moving the beam slowly gives a deeper cut with greater hemostasis, while moving rapidly gives a shallower cut with lesser hemostasis.

The power density plays a role in the depth of cutting as well. Higher power density gives a deeper cut with less hemostasis, while lower power density yields a more superficial cut with more hemostasis.

It is also possible to undermine tissue with the CO_2 laser. For this procedure the power density is somewhat reduced, but it is critical to keep the beam in the focused cutting mode rather than allowing it to slip into a defocused mode, which would vaporize the deep tissues rather than separate them cleanly. Thus, the operator's hand must follow the cutting plane precisely to keep the focal distance intact at all times. In order to achieve undermining, the hand-

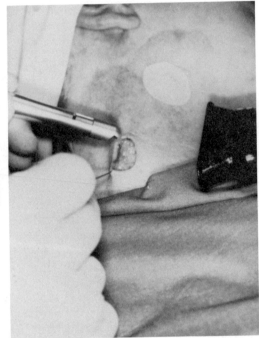

Fig 3–7.—Undermining of tissue following excision can be easily carried out with the aid of one of several angled mirrors, which can be placed at the end of the handpiece.

piece must be brought into a rather acute angle to the skin, so that the beam can be aimed under the surface. Maintaining this angle is often cumbersome, and this problem is greatly alleviated by the use of angled mirrors (Fig 3–7). These devices are supplied by many of the manufacturers and simply fit over the end of the handpiece to angle the laser beam as it exits. A 90- or 120-degree angled mirror is ideal for undermining, as it enables the operator to maintain the handpiece at a comfortable angle to the skin surface while directing the beam at an angle that is almost parallel to the surface.

After the lesion is excised, the wound bed may be lightly wiped with hydrogen peroxide on an applicator stick. This cleansing removes any surface char, which is really a very fine residue of dehydrated tissue debris. It is not at all adherent, as is the coagulum following electrosurgery. The tissue bed is now ready for immediate closure by suturing or stapling or for repair by flap or skin graft. In contrast to electrosurgery, no delay is necessary, since there is no residual layer of necrotic tissue. Wounds may also be allowed to heal by secondary intention via granulation at a rate identical to that after cold steel surgery. As was previously mentioned, the tensile strength of these wounds is identical to that of scalpel wounds by the third week postoperatively.

Specific Applications

Applications of the CO_2 laser for incisional work have included the management of rhinophyma and keloids and certain instances of Mohs' microscopically controlled excision. In treating rhinophyma (Fig 3–8) the CO_2 laser is used in both modes, cutting and vaporizing. Under local anesthesia the bulbous masses of glandular tissue are first shave-excised with the laser. There is little bleeding, and the procedure may require only a few moments. After the masses are shaved down (usually in a series of thin layers, so as not to go too deeply) the final refinements can be made by vaporizing the remaining tissue in an airbrush fashion (Fig 3–9). Thus, the nasal topography can be contoured artistically in a bloodless field and with minimal risk of the postoperative scarring that is all too common after electrosurgical procedures. Results and intraopera-

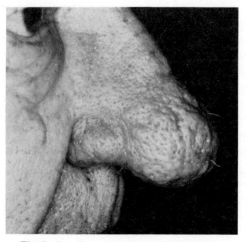

Fig 3–8.—Preoperative rhinophyma.

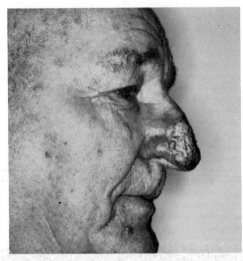

Fig 3–9.—Rhinophyma shown in Fig 3–8 immediately after CO_2 laser sculpting using both excision and vaporization.

tive comfort for both patient and surgeon far surpass those of older techniques (Fig 3–10).

The successful removal of keloids has long been a perplexing problem. We have reported the excision of recurrent or resistant keloids using the CO_2 laser in a focused cutting mode. The mass of the keloid is first shave-excised at a very high power density (Figs 3–11 and 3–12). The wound base is then palpated, and any residual fibrotic areas are identified. These areas are then excised, usually at a reduced power density. The process is repeated until no further fibrotic tissue is identifiable at the base or edges of the wound. Triamcinolone acetonide is then infiltrated throughout the field, and a pressure dressing is applied. The wound heals by secondary intention without any sutures, grafting, or other devices. Results have been highly encouraging, with over 50% of keloids healing without recurrence (Fig 3–13).

The possible explanation for this effectiveness in eliminating keloids is still being investigated. Certainly the CO_2 laser allows for a clean, atraumatic excision without the need for coagulation of vessels. No sutures are placed to cause tension and to act as foreign material. Yet there may be a more specific healing effect of the laser

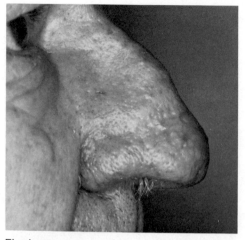

Fig 3–10.—Final appearance of healed laser sculpting of rhinophyma shown in Figs 3–8 and 3–9.

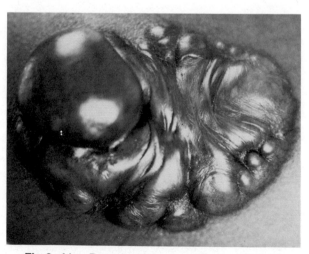

Fig 3–11.—Preoperative appearance of keloid.

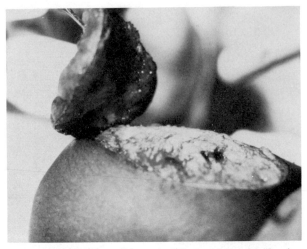

Fig 3–12.—Keloidal mass shown in Fig 3–11 is initially shave-excised with the CO_2 laser at a high power density.

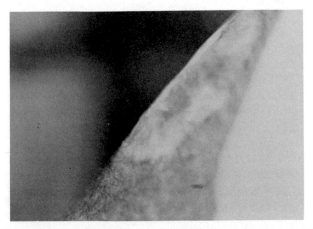

Fig 3–13.—Healed surgical site, in which there was no recurrence of the keloid shown in Figs 3–12 and 3–13.

modality. Investigators have reported that infrared laser systems used on fibroblast cultures have produced decreased levels of collagen and mucin synthesis. The CO_2 laser is in the infrared portion of the spectrum and may well exhibit similar effects on fibroblasts. This mechanism could account for the reduction in recurrent keloids following CO_2 laser surgery. It also goes along with the observed lag in tensile strength for several weeks in healing laser wounds.

The last special application of the CO_2 laser in excisional surgery is for Mohs' surgery. As we have reported, the CO_2 laser has replaced the fixed-tissue variant of the Mohs' technique in our practice. Its inherent qualities allow for the achievement of good hemostasis, excellent preservation of all histologic detail on frozen sections (Fig 3–14), tissue preservation and sparing, and the ability to excise even bone if required (Fig 3–15). Yet it is as rapid and painless as the fresh-tissue Mohs' technique.

In summary, incisional surgery with the CO_2 laser offers many advantages over cold steel or electrosurgical units. Hemostasis and lack of postoperative pain are the most readily apparent, but field sterilization, lymphatic closure, lack of excessive tissue necrosis, and power to excise even bone are other key factors.

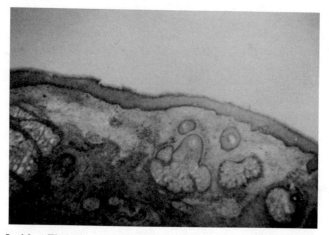

Fig 3–14.—Tissue excised with the CO_2 laser maintains its histologic integrity, making it possible to adapt this type of excision to Mohs' surgery.

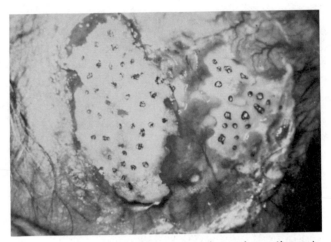

Fig 3–15.—Bone can be excised, or, as shown here, the outer table of cranial bone can be perforated to allow intertable tissue to generate granulation tissue onto the surface of the denuded bone.

VAPORIZATION

One of the attractive aspects of the CO_2 laser is its unique versatility. Not only can it be used as a precision instrument for hemostatic excision, as was described in the previous section, but it can also be used as a tool for the vaporization and ablation of a multitude of cutaneous lesions. This feat can be accomplished following relatively simple adjustments in the instrumentation. For most lasers, withdrawing the handpiece 4 to 10 in. away from the target area enables the operator to deliver an impact spot size that measures roughly 2 to 5 mm in diameter (see Fig 3–3). The net effect of this change in distance is the delivery of a much lower power density, resulting in a larger impact spot size with a much more shallow depth (see Fig 3–4). Even without changing the power output of the unit, the difference in the type of tissue damage that is caused by the defocused vs. the focused beam is quite striking. An interesting observation is that far less power output is necessary for the vaporization process than is needed for hemostatic excision. Whereas excision is most efficiently carried out at 20 to 25 W of power output, delivering 50,000 W/cm^2 of power density, vaporization is most efficiently carried out at 5 W of power output, resulting in the delivery of approximately 150 W/cm^2 of power density. Even without making the downward adjustment in the power output, the effect of defocusing the CO_2 laser beam still results in a tremendous difference in the power density delivered. A 20-W power output used for vaporization would result in the delivery of approximately 500 W/cm^2, which is considerably less than the 50,000 W/cm^2 delivered for excision.

For all practical purposes, the most important feature of laser vaporization, and yet the most difficult to become accustomed to, is the distance that the laser handpiece must be held from the target. One does not usually operate 4 to 10 in. from the operative field in scalpel surgery, and doing so with the laser is initially somewhat cumbersome. As in the excision technique, the CO_2 laser beam can be guided by use of the coaxial helium-neon laser. Most modern units are equipped with this coaxial laser, which enables the surgeon to pinpoint the area of laser impact on the target precisely. In some units, the size of the helium-neon dot on the target is roughly equivalent to the CO_2 laser impact spot size. There are various units on the market, however, in which the coaxial helium-neon dot is not related to the CO_2 impact spot size whatsoever. For this reason, it is best for the laser surgeon to become accustomed to the peculiarities of the laser with which he or she is working. The surgeon must know the impact spot size that will result from the delivery of a given power output. This knowledge can be acquired with time and experience, and it points out the need for a laser surgeon to spend ample time in practice laboratory sessions learning the fundamentals of good laser surgery.

Unlike the procedure for laser excision, the energy for laser vaporization can be delivered in a variety of ways. Initially, it may be wise for the laser surgeon to operate in the pulsed mode, delivering single short bursts of laser energy to the target site. When he is reasonably comfortable operating in this mode, the surgeon may wish to deliver multiple pulses in rapid succession, by using the rapid repeat mode. The duration of the pulses delivered is usually adjustable and is a feature on almost every available CO_2 laser unit. The experienced laser surgeon may also wish to operate in the continuous mode, delivering energy in a continuous stream, almost in an airbrush fashion. In the continuous mode, the duration of energy delivered to the target area is controlled by the surgeon with the use of the laser foot pedal. The operation of the pedal is analogous to the method of delivering electrical energy through an electrocautery or electrofulguration apparatus. The surgeon can also deliver short manually controlled pulses of energy, if desired. Manual control is particularly useful in the later passes made in treating various vascular lesions.

Once an initial pass with the laser has been made over a treatment area, the lesion usually takes on one of several appearances, depending on the amount of energy delivered and on the proximity of the handpiece to the target. With lower energies and larger impact spots, the epithelium blanches and blisters. This residue can be wiped away quite easily with a moistened cotton-tipped applicator or gauze pad. We have found hydrogen peroxide to be quite useful for cleansing treated areas immediately after the pass has been made with the laser. With higher energies and smaller impact spots, the target is more likely to take on a charred appearance almost instantaneously. This char can be cleansed from the area with hydrogen peroxide, sterile saline, or sterile water. The depth of injury one wishes to deliver for laser vaporization naturally depends on the nature of the condition being treated. (We shall consider this factor in greater detail in the next section, on specific applications for CO_2 laser vaporization.) The exact amount of laser damage deemed necessary to treat a particular condition depends to a great extent on the experience of the laser surgeon. There are no hard and fast rules, and we can merely provide guidelines, based on our observations during numerous surgical procedures. It is always in the patient's best interest for the surgeon to begin a procedure conservatively and then to make appropriate adjustments as the procedure progresses. A conservative approach costs only a small amount of time, which is inconsequential when compared to the safety and wellbeing of the patient.

One point that we should make before proceeding is that CO_2 laser vaporization is usually totally hemostatic. The operative field remains dry and bloodless. This feature alone can offer distinct advantages over alternative techniques, in which bleeding may be prominent. Finally, because CO_2 laser vaporization has been known to seal off nerve endings, preventing the release of the transmitters that are necessary for pain sensation, the postoperative course is usually painless. Occasional burning pain may be present for several hours immediately following the procedure, and there may be tenderness during wound care, but other discomfort is quite rare.

Specific Applications

The CO_2 laser is a surgical instrument. As such, it can be used at the discretion of the surgeon to excise or vaporize any cutaneous lesions. While it does not always offer unique or distinct advantages over more conventional procedures, there are a variety of cutaneous lesions for which CO_2 laser vaporization is, without question, superior to other modalities. Experience alone will help delineate those conditions for which CO_2 laser vaporization is the treatment of choice. The following sections discuss several conditions for which CO_2 laser vaporization has already been demonstrated to be uniquely suited. Though the technique is basically the same (i.e., vaporization, cleansing of char, vaporization, and so on), each condition has certain unique characteristics with which the cutaneous laser surgeon should be familiar.

EPIDERMAL NEVI—Verrucous epidermal nevi are characteristic in appearance (Fig 3–16) and uniformly difficult to treat. In order to achieve acceptable cosmetic results, the surgeon may be faced with the problem of recurrence. Excision, cryosurgery, and dermabrasion have all been variably successful in treating epidermal nevi. CO_2 laser vaporization is also useful, but the final cosmetic result should always be considered. For smaller, linear lesions, excision resulting in a fine linear scar is always preferable to the broader atrophic or hypertrophic scars resulting from cryosurgery, dermabrasion, or laser vaporization. For broader lesions appearing on ventral surfaces or glabrous skin, superficial cryosurgery may offer distinct advantages in achieving a good cosmetic result. We have found that CO_2 laser vaporization is most effective in treating epidermal nevi of the head and neck and dorsal hair-bearing areas, where it offers the prospect of exceptionally good cosmetic results. It may also be the best method for use in intertriginous areas, where the cosmetic result is less important but where it offers distinct advantages because it minimizes scarring and stricture.

Once evaluation has been made and the alternatives have been

Fig 3–16.—Typical appearance of verrucous epidermal nevus.

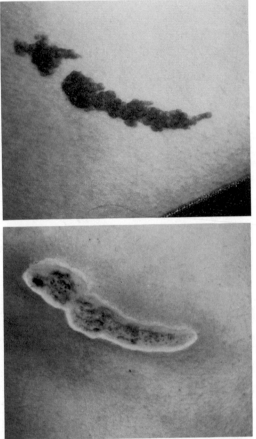

Fig 3–17.—Characteristic "inside of orange peel" appearance of tissue immediately following CO_2 laser vaporization of epidermal nevus shown in Fig 3–16.

Fig 3–18.—Final appearance of scar resulting from vaporization of epidermal nevus shown in Figs 3–16 and 3–17. In this instance, no cosmetic advantage was seen over what might have been expected by cold steel excision.

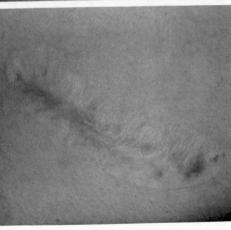

considered, the following guidelines may be employed if CO_2 laser vaporization has been decided on as the appropriate procedure. A test area should be selected for treatment. It should be representative of the overall lesion and in an area that can be hidden, if possible, in case unsightly scarring occurs instead of the good cosmetic result desired.

The test area is prepared as for any surgical procedure, and local anesthesia is administered. Occasionally, it may be helpful to outline the anesthetized area to be treated with brilliant green or gentian violet dye. An appropriate power setting (e.g., 5 W) is selected, and vaporization proceeds steadily over the test area. It is often best to treat the perimeter of the test area first, to assure complete anesthesia, and then to proceed with the remainder of the field. Once the entire area has been treated, the char is cleansed from the area, and the procedure is repeated as many times as necessary to ablate the nevus. Normally, vaporized tissue has the appearance of the inside of an orange peel (Fig 3–17). Epidermal nevus tissue is slightly darker in color and is not too difficult to distinguish from uninvolved, normal tissue. The use of a 2.5-power (or greater) magnifying loupe may be of benefit in distinguishing involved from uninvolved tissue, especially in the later stages of surgery. Usually, three to four passes over the area are required for ablation of these lesions, but this number may be higher depending on the power and spot size of the laser and the thickness and location of the lesion.

Once the area has been treated, it is cleansed and dressed appropriately. Reepithelialization should be complete in two to four weeks, depending on the size and location of the spot. If hypertrophic scarring occurs, it should appear within 12 weeks. For this reason, the final decision on whether or not to proceed with laser ablation is best made three months after treating the test patch.

If the desired result is achieved, removal of the remainder of the lesion can then begin. This removal is often best carried out in a staged fashion. The appropriate size of the areas to be treated depends on their location and on other factors such as the amount of local anesthesia that can be safely delivered. The time interval between procedures should be at least the length of time it takes for the earlier wounds to reepithelialize but is left to the discretion of the physician. At the early stages of treatment, a conservative approach is paramount (Fig 3–18).

DECORATIVE OR TRAUMATIC TATTOOS—Although numerous methods of tattoo removal are available, many physicians feel that CO_2 laser vaporization is the treatment of choice. If a tattoo cannot be excised with a fine linear scar as the final result, then laser ablation may very well be the preferred treatment modality.

In general, professional tattoos are easier to remove than amateur tattoos, because of the uniform depth of the pigment. The mid-chest, ventral forearm, and deltoid areas are highly troublesome to treat, in that hypertrophic scarring is common and often unavoidable. Tattoos that have been present for at least several years are also often more difficult to remove, because of pigment migration to the deeper dermis.

With these points in mind, preparation, outline, and anesthesia of the area are carried out as for epidermal nevi. It is often prudent to outline the tattoo in an irregular or geometric shape, so as not to leave the patient with a scar in the same shape as the original tattoo. The patient may wish to have a test area done first, but because many tattoo patients don't return for treatment, it is often best

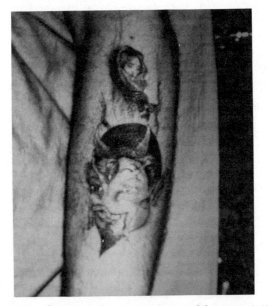

Fig 3–19.—Preoperative appearance of forearm tattoo.

simply to treat the area totally or to begin removal without benefit of a test spot (Fig 3–19).

Vaporization proceeds as described for epidermal nevi, usually at 5 W. The tattoo becomes quite brilliant after the initial pass, and the uninvolved skin again resembles the inside of an orange peel. By the third pass, the tattoo pigment begins to fade, and the surgeon can then concentrate on the pigment alone, without treating the uninvolved adjacent tissue. Occasionally, it is necessary to adopt a smaller spot size (i.e., to bring the laser into slightly better focus) to achieve good pigment removal. Many laser surgeons stop after completing four to six passes (Fig 3–20), since much of residual pigmentation will "wash out" as granulation occurs. Residual pigment that persists can then be revaporized at a later date. Our practice is to remove all but perhaps a trace of the pigment, eliminating the need for further surgery. The choice of how much pigment to leave is a matter of individual preference, and neither method is clearly supe-

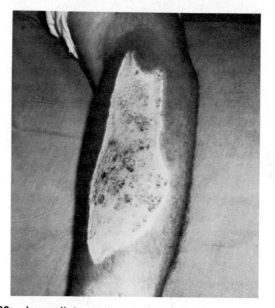

Fig 3–20.—Immediate postoperative appearance of site at which tattoo shown in Fig 3–19 was vaporized. All traces of pigment were removed in this case. Dark areas in the center of the wound represent residual tissue char.

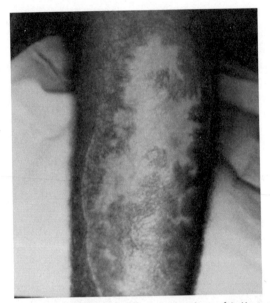

Fig 3–21.—Final healed result of vaporization of tattoo shown in Figs 3–19 and 3–20. Scar is soft, flat, and supple. There is some hair growth, and repigmentation is almost complete.

rior. Most tattoo patients, however, prefer that all the pigment be removed and also prefer that this be done in as few stages as possible (Fig 3–21).

Daily wound care is extremely important for the tattoo patient. Our usual practice is to instruct the patient to cleanse the wound daily with hydrogen peroxide and then to apply a thin coat of Polysporin ointment and cover it with an occlusive Telfa-type dressing. A more thorough discussion of wound care can be found at the end of this chapter.

PORT-WINE STAINS—Laser therapy is virtually the only choice for treatment of port-wine stains. The argon laser is probably the most widely used for this condition, but there is some controversy regarding laser therapy in this area. In theory, the argon laser treats port-wine stains by selectively sealing off vessels filled with red blood cells, which maximally absorb the complementary argon light energy. The CO_2 laser is thought to work by thermally sealing off vessels in a nonselective fashion, but with minimal thermal damage to surrounding structures. Current histologic studies seem to show that nonspecific thermal damage is the active event for both argon and CO_2 laser therapy, with the resulting healing occurring in clinically and histologically identical fashion. Some more recent work suggests that argon laser therapy at very low fluence may indeed show the theorized specificity, but this premise has not been adequately borne out.

Another area of controversy also exists. Some laser surgeons believe that lighter port-wine stains respond best to CO_2 vaporization while darker ones do best with argon ablation. Other surgeons believe that darker port-wine stains respond well to either laser, while lighter ones are less likely to respond favorably.

The answers to these controversies are simply not known at this time. Our approach is to test prospective patients with both lasers and evaluate the results after three months. Patient and physician input are both used to determine how to proceed. We are finding that it is simply not possible to predict beforehand with any degree of accuracy which port-wine stains will respond best to which laser. Perhaps, as has been suggested, the key to this problem lies in the "blanchability" of the lesion (that is, how well a lesion blanches on diascopy).

Vaporization with the CO_2 laser proceeds as described previously, with selection of an appropriate and representative test site, preparation, outline, and anesthesia. Epinephrine may be used to prolong the anesthesia without impairing the progress of the CO_2 laser surgery, unlike argon laser surgery. The initial pass can be made at 5 W, causing the tissue to blanch and blister. The damaged epithelium is then cleansed away with a damp sponge, and a second pass is made. Two or three passes are usually sufficient to ablate the majority of the vessels. Once again, a 2.5-power magnifying loupe may be quite helpful in examining the wound. Residual vessels are vaporized by bringing the laser into slightly sharper focus, as was described for tattoos. When ablation is completed, the wound should have the appearance of the inside of an orange peel. Darker port-wine stains, when treated in this fashion, have a similar appearance but look "peppered" or "stepped on" because of the black color of the thermally thrombosed vessels (Figs 3–22 to 3–24).

Daily wound care instructions should be outlined for the pa-

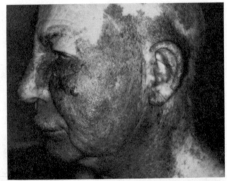

Fig 3–22.—Dark, verrucous port-wine stain preoperatively.

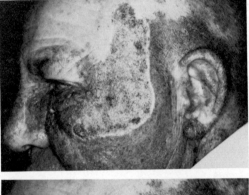

Fig 3–23.—"Inside of orange peel" appearance of wound immediately after CO_2 laser vaporization of port-wine stain shown in Fig 3–22.

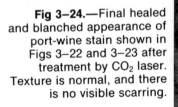

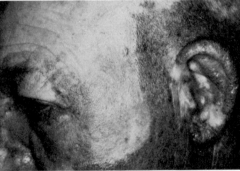

Fig 3–24.—Final healed and blanched appearance of port-wine stain shown in Figs 3–22 and 3–23 after treatment by CO_2 laser. Texture is normal, and there is no visible scarring.

tient, and the patient is seen again after reepithelialization, usually in four to six weeks. A decision on whether or not to proceed with the total ablation should not be made for at least three months. In addition to the scarring that may occur within 12 weeks, both CO_2- and argon-treated wounds are subject to a delayed blanch phenomenon, in which blanching of the lesion may not actually occur for up to one year following laser surgery.

When the decision has been made to proceed with CO_2 laser vaporization, then a staged removal is planned, as has been discussed previously. Treatment then proceeds in the same fashion already described for vaporization of the test area.

Verruca Vulgaris—Although several methods exist for the treatment of recalcitrant warts, all are doomed to a certain amount of failure. The CO_2 laser may offer advantages over the other methods in several respects. The wounds from CO_2 laser vaporization of warts are, for the most part, virtually painless. The scarring is minimized in these areas, and normal sensation of the fingers is usually not compromised. In addition, periungual and subungual warts can often be treated without the need for nail avulsion, since the laser can vaporize the overlying nail and reach the involved nail bed. While the choice of method may end up being based on personal preference, CO_2 laser vaporization certainly has been shown to be effective.

Before proceeding with the vaporization of warts, it is frequently beneficial to soak the area in a warm, soapy solution for 15 to 20 minutes. This soaking seems to aid in the progress of the laser vaporization. Once the area has been soaked, cleaned, and prepared, local or regional anesthesia is administered. Carbon dioxide laser vaporization then proceeds in the manner previously outlined for other lesions. It may be necessary, and is often beneficial, to increase the power output of the laser to 20 to 25 W for verrucal vaporization. The adjustment in power output seems to enhance the effectiveness of laser vaporization for this particular type of lesion. As the vaporization is carried out, wart tissue has a tendency to bubble in a very characteristic fashion. Because the surrounding normal tissue does not behave in this way, the surgeon is usually able to visualize the necessary extent of laser vaporization. When dealing with hyperkeratotic surfaces, such as the plantar aspect of the foot, repeat passes may be necessary for complete lesion removal. After several passes have been made, the main bulk of hyperkeratotic lesion is often freed when the area is cleaned between passes. A red and sometimes bleeding base is revealed, which can then be vaporized further. A curet may be handy for removing thick char or stubborn residue left from the laser vaporization.

For larger verrucae, a combination of excision and vaporization is occasionally necessary for complete, adequate, and efficient wart removal. Once the lesion has been adequately removed to the satisfaction of the laser surgeon, the wound is cleaned and dressed appropriately and is allowed to reepithelialize by secondary intention. As with warts treated by other methods, incubating verrucae may sometimes become apparent following laser vaporization. When such lesions do appear, they should be vaporized at the time of the follow-up visit. This treatment reduces the chance of further spread of the wart virus.

ADDITIONAL APPLICATIONS—As we already mentioned, CO_2 laser vaporization offers unique and distinct advantages over conventional methods of surgery in many instances. These advantages may not always be clear-cut, but they are present nevertheless. Lichen sclerosus et atrophicus, especially in the form of balanitis xerotica obliterans, has been shown to be very effectively treated with CO_2 laser vaporization (Figs 3–25 to 3–27). Symptoms have completely disappeared in patients treated in this fashion. Superficial basal cell carcinoma and Bowen's disease can likewise be easily treated with this modality. Adnexal tumors and telangiectasias also respond to this type of therapy. When these lesions are present in great numbers, the treatment of choice may very well be CO_2 laser-"brasion," which has the same net effect as dermabrasion, but in a totally bloodless fashion. This same type of bloodless cosmetic surgery can be applied to bulbous rhinophyma, as was discussed in the section on laser excision. As we noted, a combination of excision and vaporization with the CO_2 laser can be employed to sculpt a more normal-appearing nose when sebaceous hyperplasia is present in rhinophyma (see Figs 3–8 to 3–10). The advantages of using the laser during this procedure are hemostasis and a painless postoperative course. The results are very gratifying and compare favorably to those achieved with other modalities.

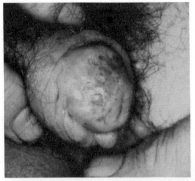

Fig 3–25.—Balanitis xerotica obliterans preoperatively.

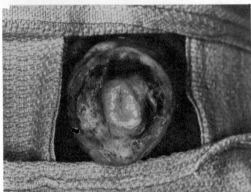

Fig 3–26.—Immediate postoperative appearance of laser-treated balanitis xerotica obliterans, allowing reepithelialization from uninvolved adjacent tissue (same patient as in Fig 3–25).

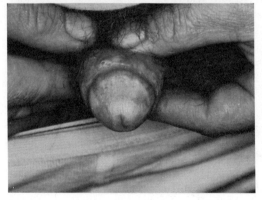

Fig 3–27.—Final result of laser-treated balanitis xerotica obliterans after uneventful postoperative course. Tissue reaction is minimal after CO_2 laser treatment, so edema and fibrotic stricture do not occur (same patient as in Figs 3–25 and 3–26).

It goes without saying that this list of lesions that can be treated by CO_2 laser vaporization is only a partial one. Virtually any lesion can be treated by this method, and, if readily available, the CO_2 laser certainly offers an attractive alternative to conventional modes of therapy.

Wound Care

Although postoperative wound care is a controversial subject, there is reason to believe that proper wound care benefits the patient by increasing the chance of a good to excellent cosmetic result. Our wound care procedure is basically the same for most applications of CO_2 laser vaporization. Once the surgery has been completed, the wound is carefully cleaned with sterile water, sterile saline, a surgical scrub, or, as is our preference, hydrogen peroxide. The entire wound is then covered with an occlusive antibacterial ointment, and a nonstick Telfa dressing is applied directly over the ointment, followed by a rolled gauze dressing. When possible, an attempt is made to avoid direct contact between tape and skin. When it is not possible to avoid contact, a hypoallergenic type of adhesive should be employed, if available. The patient is instructed to clean the wound daily with either a surgical scrub or hydrogen peroxide and to follow this cleansing with the application of the antibacterial ointment and nonstick dressing. We have found that some of the newer occlusive dressings that are commercially available (e.g., Vigilon and Duoderm) may offer distinct advantages by promoting faster wound healing and by decreasing the tendency to form unsightly scars. We have been favorably impressed with the preliminary use of these materials in many of our patients who have undergone vaporization. It is possible that they may become the dressings of choice following CO_2 laser surgery.

Once healing has progressed so that reepithelialization is complete, occlusive dressings are no longer necessary. At this point, except for lesions of an infective nature (such as verruca vulgaris), we often instruct the patient to begin applying a moderately potent steroid ointment twice daily. Although the efficacy of this procedure still remains questionable, we believe that the use of a steroid ointment at this stage of healing may very well reduce the chance of hypertrophic scarring. When a steroid ointment is used prior to reepithelialization, it retards the progress of wound healing and may delay reepithelialization by as much as several months. Pressure dressings, while quite beneficial, may likewise retard reepithelialization. If pressure dressings are to be employed, it may be prudent to delay their use until reepithelialization is complete. The application of topical steroids, pressure dressings, or both may then proceed for the remainder of the 12-week postoperative period.

Pain has been a rare complication of CO_2 laser vaporization, but it has occurred on occasion. Mild analgesia is sometimes required, and changes in wound care may be advisable. Application of topical or viscous anesthetic agents such as lidocaine hydrochloride (Xylocaine) may offer immediate but temporary relief. Usually, temporary relief is all that is necessary, since discomfort becomes less of a problem as wound healing is allowed to continue.

DISCUSSION

Although CO_2 laser excision and vaporization are fairly new modalities for the cutaneous surgeon, their use is ever growing. There is no question that changes in techniques and advances in technology will alter the ways in which these procedures can be carried out. For the time being, however, it is hoped that the techniques outlined here offer insight to the beginning laser surgeon on how to proceed with safe and successful CO_2 laser surgery.

BIBLIOGRAPHY

Apfelberg, D., et al. Histology of port-wine stains following argon laser treatment. *Br. J. Plast. Surg.* 32:232–237, 1979.
Bailin, P. L., and Wheeland, R. G. Carbon dioxide (CO_2) laser perforation of exposed bone to stimulate granulation tissue. *Plast. Reconstr. Surg.* 75(6):898–902, 1985.
Bailin, P. L.; Ratz, J. L.; and Levine, H. L. Removal of tattoos by CO_2 laser. *J. Dermatol. Surg. Oncol.* 6:977–1001, 1980.
Bailin, P. L.; Ratz, J. L.; and Lutz-Nagey, L. CO_2 laser modification of Mohs' surgery. *J. Dermatol. Surg. Oncol.* 7:621–623, 1981.
Buecker, J. W.; Ratz, J. L.; and Richfield, D. Histology of CO_2 laser treatment of port-wine stains. *J. Am. Acad. Dermatol.* 10:1014–1019, 1984.

104   P. L. BAILIN, J. L. RATZ

Finley, J., et al. Healing of port-wine stains after argon laser therapy. *Arch. Dermatol.* 117:486–489, 1981.

Gilchrest, B.; Rosen, G.; and Noe, J. Chilling port-wine stains improves the response to argon laser therapy. *Plast. Reconstr. Surg.* 69:278–283, 1982.

Levine, H. L., and Bailin, P. L. CO_2 laser treatment of cutaneous tattoos and angiomas. *Arch. Otolaryngol.* 108(4):236–238, 1983.

McBurney, E. I. Carbon dioxide laser surgery of dermatologic lesions. *South. Med. J.* 71:795–797, 1978.

Noe, J., et al. Port-wine stains and the response to argon laser therapy: successful treatment and the predictive role of color, age, and biopsy. *Plast. Reconstr. Surg.* 65:130–136, 1980.

Ratz, J. L. CO_2 laser for the treatment of balanitis xerotica obliterans. *J. Am. Acad. Dermatol.* 10(5):925–928, 1984.

Ratz, J. L., and Luu, S. T. CO_2 laser vs. dermabrasion for reduction of rhinophyma (manuscript in progress).

Ratz, J. L.; Bailin, P. L.; and Levine, H. L. CO_2 laser treatment of port-wine stains: a preliminary report. *J. Dermatol. Surg. Oncol.* 8:1039–1044, 1982.

Read, R., and Muller, S. Tattoo removal by CO_2 laser dermabrasion. *Plast. Reconstr. Surg.* 65:717–728, 1980.

Rosenberg, S. K., et al. Continuous way CO_2 treatment of balanitis xerotica obliterans. *Urology* 19(5):539–541, 1982.

Wheeland, R. G., and Bailin, P. L. Dermatologic applications of the argon and carbon dioxide (CO_2) laser. *Current Concepts in Skin Disorders* 5:5–11, 1984.

Wheeland, R. G., and Bailin, P. L. Scalp reduction surgery with the carbon dioxide (CO_2) laser. *J. Dermatol. Surg. Oncol.* 10:565–569, 1984.

Wheeland, R. G.; Bailin, P. L.; and Kronberg, E. Carbon dioxide (CO_2) laser vaporization for the treatment of multiple trichoepitheliomata. *J. Dermatol. Surg. Oncol.* 10:470–475, 1984.

4

OTHER LASERS IN DERMATOLOGY: THE PAST AND THE FUTURE

CHRISTOPHER R. SHEA, M.D.

OON TIAN TAN, M.D.

JOHN A. PARRISH, M.D.

THIS CHAPTER reviews work on the cutaneous effects of lasers other than the argon and carbon dioxide (CO_2) lasers. At present, the lasers reviewed here are not much used in clinical dermatology. While some of these instruments are mainly of historical interest, others are useful in research, and some will likely become important clinical tools in the near future. The chapter concludes with a perspective on laser phototherapy and a look at possible future directions in research and development.

Table 4–1 gives an overview of the principal features of the lasers discussed in this chapter.

TABLE 4–1.—Summary of Possible Applications of Lesser-Used Lasers

LASER	WAVELENGTH (NM)	POSSIBLE THERAPEUTIC APPLICATIONS IN DERMATOLOGY
Ruby	694	Nevi; cancer; port-wine hemangioma; tattoo removal
Neodymium	1,060	Surgical hemostasis; cancer; keloids
Nitrogen	337	Focal topical psoralen ultraviolet A (PUVA) photochemotherapy
Tunable dye	200–700	Port-wine hemangioma; photoradiation therapy of cancer; tattoo removal
Copper vapor	578	(Research tool)
Excimer	157; 193; 248; 308; 351	Ablation of growths; incisions in plastic surgery

RUBY LASER

Biomedical applications of lasers began with the ruby laser. In this instrument, the active medium is a ruby crystal infused with chromium ion (Cr^{3+}), which is emitted at 694.3 nm. The pulse duration is nominally around 1 msec, but this figure actually represents a train of pulses on the order of 1 μsec each. Alternatively, the ruby laser can be operated in the Q-switched mode, with a single defined pulse of about 10 to 50 nsec.

The fundamental studies of Goldman and colleagues involved comparisons between white and black human volunteers and between albino and pigmented rabbits. They found that the necrotic and inflammatory reactions of skin to the ruby laser were melanin dependent; the studies demonstrated that the threshold for these effects could be lowered by pigmenting the skin with soot or paint. Goldman also recognized that both power density (irradiance) and energy density (dose) are important variables that affect the biologic response to lasers. Subsequently, his laboratory reported the first delivery of ruby laser beams to skin via fiberoptics.

Ruby laser irradiation causes both dermal and epidermal damage. Superficial splitting of the stratum corneum is produced at low doses. At higher doses the effect proceeds to epidermal dyskeratosis, vacuolation, and pyknosis; dermal and epidermal edema; coagulation of collagen; perivascular lymphocytic and histiocytic infiltrate; and a variable degree of vascular damage.

The ruby laser was the first laser used to treat port-wine hemangioma. Doses of 50 joules/cm^2 caused immediate necrosis. Reepithelialization followed an inflammatory phase, with the eventual formation of a dense cicatrix that spared the skin appendages. By six months after treatment, blood vessels in irradiated skin were scarce and compressed, and the port-wine stain appeared blanched. Although this treatment gave satisfactory cosmetic results, the relatively nonselective absorption of red light by blood and melanin caused extensive damage to both epidermal and dermal structures.

As early as 1964 the ruby laser was used to treat skin cancer in dosages that ranged from 100 to 7,800 joules/cm^2. Doses that were sufficient to cause severe thermal injury caused relatively more local destruction in melanoma, hemorrhagic Kaposi's sarcoma, and pigmented basal cell carcinoma than in mycosis fungoides, Bowen's disease, or nonpigmented basal cell carcinoma. While no long-term follow-up studies were performed, local recurrences were noted. The ruby laser is still sometimes used to treat primary melanoma, but its use is controversial in comparison to the more widely used primary surgical approaches. Ohshiro and Maruyama have used ruby and argon laser systems to treat more than 4,000 cases of pigmented nevi; the ruby laser gave superior cosmetic results when the lesions were relatively superficial. The ruby laser has also been used successfully to treat the oral hypermelanosis of Peutz-Jeghers syndrome.

Q-switched ruby lasers can be used to lighten decorative tattoos, as can many other lasers, including argon, CO_2, Nd-YAG, and tunable dye lasers. Regardless of the color of the tattoo pigment or the laser wavelength employed, laser treatment of tattoos produces thermally induced necrosis, followed by sloughing and fibrosis. The cosmetic result thus primarily reflects a host response to a thermal insult (slough and bury) rather than a particular photochemical reaction of the tattoo to light. The question of how the variables can be manipulated to alter these host responses is largely unexplored.

Although the ruby laser has found many applications in dermatology, it has been superceded by other systems that offer more useful wavelengths. The effects of the ruby laser on the skin are rather nonselective, because its wavelength of 694 nm falls within the 600 to 1,200 nm therapeutic window, a range that is absorbed relatively weakly by endogenous pigments. By the same token, however, the ruby laser may find new applications as schemes are developed for targeting tissues with exogenous chromophores that can absorb radiation at wavelengths that fall within this window. In one such experiment, intravenous injection of the albumin-bound dye indocyanine green in rabbits caused a threefold enhancement of ruby laser efficiency in producing cutaneous purpura.

Nd-YAG LASER

In the neodymium–yttrium-aluminum-garnet (Nd-YAG) laser the active medium is neodymium, added as a dopant to an yttrium-aluminum-garnet crystal; a related laser uses neodymium-doped glass. The radiation is in the near-infrared (1.06-μm wavelength) range and can be emitted in pulses or in a continuous wave. Unlike the CO_2 laser, which emits radiation in the far-infrared (10.6-μm wavelength) range, the energy of the Nd-YAG laser is not absorbed by water, penetrates deeply into tissue (about 37% of the radiation incident on the skin reaches a depth of 2 mm), and is widely scattered within the dermis, thereby exposing a large volume of tissue. The result is often widespread coagulation necrosis and hemostasis. Because of its hemostatic capability, the Nd-YAG laser is used in some cold-steel surgical procedures.

In 1973 Goldman and colleagues reported success in treating tattoos, port-wine hemangiomas, blue rubber bleb nevus, basal cell carcinoma, and squamous cell carcinoma with high-intensity Nd-YAG lasers. Good hemostasis was effected, even in highly vascular lesions, in contrast to the poor hemostasis seen with CO_2 laser surgery. Another advantage of the Nd-YAG over the CO_2 laser is its ability to be directed through fiberoptics.

Recently, the continuous-wave Nd-YAG laser has been used successfully in eight patients to treat keloids that had been refractory to steroid injection and excision. These results contrast with the reported poor response of keloids to argon and CO_2 laser irradiation. The deep penetration of the Nd-YAG radiation may be responsible for its efficacy in this condition. Basic studies provide a rationale for the use of this laser in flattening keloids. Nd-YAG irradiation of human fibroblasts in vitro caused decreased collagen synthesis, whereas heating by an incandescent lamp did not have this effect. Irradiation of pig skin in vivo caused a reduction in total collagen content 60 days after treatment, reflecting decreased synthesis rather than increased degradation, while a thermal treatment by electrocautery had no such effect on collagen metabolism. Heating under two different conditions may cause very different results, however; rate-process models of thermal damage predict that the total time-temperature history of the tissue determines the final effect. More work is therefore needed to determine if these results reflect a nonthermal mechanism.

The Nd-YAG laser has been used extensively in the Soviet Union to treat cutaneous neoplasms. Following animal studies, Wagner and associates irradiated benign and malignant tumors of the skin with a pulsed Nd-glass laser. In 516 cases of carcinoma of the skin (histologic findings unspecified), there were no reported recurrences; the mean follow-up time appears to have been about three years. In an expanded series of 79 melanoma patients, two local recurrences were noted after laser treatment. Of the 70 melanoma patients with no palpable metastases before treatment, 15 (21.4%) had subsequent development of metastases in regional nodes, subcutaneous fat, or viscera. Of the 34 patients followed for five or more years after laser treatment began, 25 (73.5%) continued to survive free of disease. These studies give no details on the extent of workup for metastasis or on the protocol for follow-up study, and statistical interpretation is completely absent. Furthermore, the diagnosis of melanoma was made cytologically by means of touch preparations or thin-needle aspiration, so that histologic distinctions of tumor type are lacking.

One concern raised by this mode of therapy is whether cancer may be spread iatrogenically by the high energy of the laser pulse. Because of their softness and high optical absorbance, melanomas tend to explode or vaporize after exposure to Nd-YAG laser pulses, while harder tumors such as sarcomas and breast carcinomas transmit the absorbed energy as kinetic propulsion. Hoye and colleagues were able to grow melanoma implants from viable cells that had been shot several meters from the impact site of the pulsed Nd-YAG laser, using huge power densities of 10^8 W/cm^2 and energy densities of up to 10^6 joules/cm^2. The clinical relevance of these results is unclear. It is unknown whether any viable tumor cells could traverse the zone of coagulation around the impact site and then metastasize by hematogenous or lymphatic spread. In their treatment of malignant melanoma with the Nd-YAG laser, the Soviet authors irradiated an outer ring of normal tissue before treating the tumor, in order to reduce the risk of dissemination.

A serious disadvantage of laser treatment of primary melanoma is that it destroys the pathologic specimen, so that microstaging and checking the margins for malignant cells are impossible. Since excision is both diagnostic and potentially curative, it is hard to justify substituting a procedure that is only potentially curative. Furthermore, needling a melanoma for diagnostic purposes may risk spreading it.

A recent study in mice demonstrated that the effect of the Nd-YAG laser on the growth rate of experimental breast adenocarcinomas implanted into skin is energy density dependent. Substantial tumor destruction was seen at energy doses that caused no immediate necrosis or charring; this finding is consistent with the increased sensitivity of cancer cells to moderate hyperthermia.

The Nd-YAG laser may eventually prove useful in treating skin cancer; more basic studies and much better controlled clinical trials are needed before it can be widely accepted for this application.

NITROGEN LASER

The nitrogen (N_2) laser emits pulses of radiation at a wavelength of 337.1 nm, which falls within the long-wave ultraviolet (UV-A) region (320 to 400 nm). Its monochromaticity and power have made it useful in research on the erythemal and pigmentary responses of human skin to UV-A. Using a source emitting 10-nsec pulses at a repetition rate of between 1 and 500 pulses per second, the threshold for delayed erythema and pigmentation in fair-skinned white subjects averaged about 20 joules/cm². This threshold is comparable to reported values arrived at by using nonlaser UV-A radiation sources. Furthermore, this value did not vary significantly within individual subjects over a threefold range of peak irradiance. In contrast, immediate erythema was irradiance dependent, occurring only above 20 mW/cm² or above 100 pulses per second. This finding suggests that immediate erythema is at least partially a thermal effect; a local temperature rise was noted during the high-irradiance exposures.

The pulsed N_2 laser is primarily a research tool and has not as yet found wide clinical application. Preliminary studies have shown the N_2 laser to be a convenient but expensive method for treating small skin lesions (such as warts) photosensitized with topically applied psoralens. The N_2 laser can also be used to pump a tunable dye laser with variable wavelength output, and in this role it has more clinical promise.

TUNABLE DYE LASERS

The active medium in tunable dye lasers is a liquid dye that lases by fluorescence after optic pumping by a flash lamp or by another laser (e.g., an N_2 or argon laser). Depending on the pumping apparatus used, the output may be pulsed or in a continuous wave. This output can then be tuned over a wide range of wavelengths by changing the dye and certain other operating parameters. As research tools tunable dye lasers have been used to generate photobiologic action spectra and for in vitro studies of photochemistry. They are now also beginning to be used clinically, and their versatility gives them unique advantages in this area.

In general, the monochromatic aspects of lasers have not been crucial to their medical applications, since most biologic absorbance spectra are broad and overlapping, and many wavelengths may have roughly equivalent effects. It is possible, however, to exploit the monochromaticity of lasers, by using wavelengths that are especially well absorbed by pigments distributed nonuniformly in tissue.

For example, a pulsed dye laser can be tuned so as to produce highly selective vascular damage. To produce this effect, the laser is tuned to a wavelength of 577 nm, which corresponds to the α band of oxyhemoglobin. This wavelength penetrates substantially to the depth of the dermal blood vessels and is subject to little interfering absorption by melanin. The duration of exposure is chosen by considering the thermal relaxation time of blood vessels, modeled as cylinders with the thermal properties of water. Based on these calculations, pulses with a duration of 1 to 20 msec should be on the order of the thermal relaxation time of blood vessels with a diameter of 50 μm. It was therefore predicted that by using pulses shorter than 1 msec, the heating would be effectively confined to these small dermal vessels. In this approach, known as selective photothermolysis, a target is heated to a temperature above the threshold for irreversible damage; as the heat dissipates, the surrounding tissue is also heated by conduction, but to a temperature below the critical threshold (Fig 4–1).

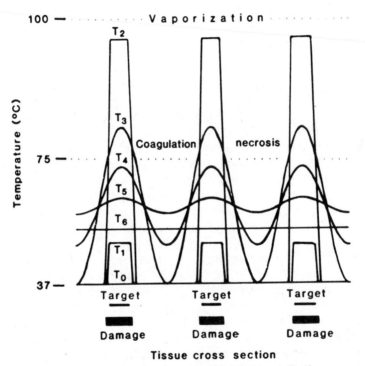

Fig 4–1.—Schematic temperature profiles during selective photothermolysis: T_0, before laser exposure (uniform body temperature); T_1, during laser exposure (selective rapid target healing); T_2, at the end of laser exposure (targets irreversibly damaged); T_3, one thermal relaxation time after laser pulse (targets cooling, surrounding tissue warming); T_4, two thermal relaxation times after laser pulse; T_5, five thermal relaxation times after laser pulse; and T_6, tissue slowly returning to ambient thermal equilibrium. (From *Science* 220:521, 1983. Used by permission.)

The basic theory of selective photothermolysis was validated in experiments on human volunteers whose skin was irradiated with 300-nsec pulses at 577 nm and at energy densities from 0.5 to 5 joules/cm^2. Grossly, purpura occurred in white subjects at 2 to 3 joules/cm^2. Specific vascular effects were seen histologically: erythrocyte aggregation ensued immediately, sometimes with rupture of vessels, and an acute necrotizing vasculitis and perivasculitis appeared in the upper dermis by 48 hours after exposure (Fig 4−2). Electron micrographs show erythrocyte aggregation at 1.5 μsec pulse duration, with necrosis of endothelial cells and pericytes but with no major damage to perivascular collagen, histiocytes, mast cells, or fibroblasts (Figs 4−3 and 4−4). As the pulse duration was increased, so was the energy density necessary to reach the purpura threshold; there was also a concomitant increase in the zone of damage surrounding the "internal heater," hemoglobin. Purpura did not occur when the laser was tuned to 590 nm; the effect was thus a highly sensitive function of wavelength.

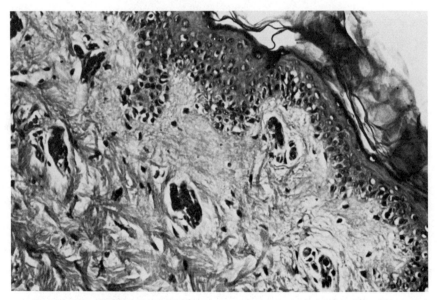

Fig 4−2.—Agglutinated red blood cells occluding the lumina of several vessels in the horizontal subpapillary plexus, following experimental selective photothermolysis.

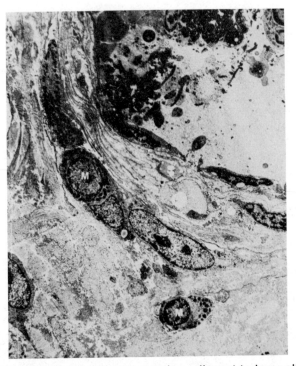

Fig 4–3.—Endothelial cell degeneration adjacent to laser-altered erythrocytes. Note intact perivascular collagen bundles and mast cells (M).

In contrast to the dye laser's selective vascular effects, the argon laser at threshold doses causes widespread coagulative necrosis of the epidermis and of the dermal collagen, as well as vascular damage. The argon laser's emission lines lie between the Soret absorption band of oxyhemoglobin at 418 nm and the β band at 542 nm; it is therefore not optically ideal for causing selective damage to targets bearing oxyhemoglobin.

When the skin was cooled to 10 C before irradiation with 300-nsec pulses at 577 nm, the mean threshold energy density for purpura increased; the threshold was not changed, however, when the blood perfusion of the skin was altered by pressure, intradermal epinephrine injection, or prior UV-B treatment. These data are consistent with intravascular microvaporization as the mechanism of purpura formation.

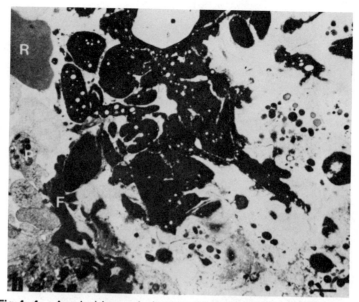

Fig 4–4.—Ameboid morphology and increased electron density of laser-altered erythrocytes, with formation of vacuoles (80 nm in diameter) within erythrocytes. *F*, fibroblast; *R*, red blood cell; *P*, platelet.

After irradiating exposed hamster cheek pouches with the same pulsed dye laser at 577 nm, a sequence of microscopic changes occurred that were dependent on energy density; these changes ranged from brown discoloration to temporary hemostasis to permanent hemostasis to rupture. The threshold for these effects varied directly with the vessel diameter. Cooling the cheek pouch to 8 C before irradiation increased the energy threshold for all of these effects.

Epidermal pigmentation can limit the vascular selectivity of the dye laser tuned to 577 nm. In subjects whose pigmentation spanned the range from vitiligo to dark black (skin types I to VI, respectively), the threshold dose for purpura was lower for fair-skinned subjects; it was impossible to produce purpura in the darkest-skinned subjects. Skin types I to IV demonstrated selective vascular changes, while epidermal damage predominated in skin types V and VI (Figs 4–5 and 4–6).

The finding that blood vessels can be selectively damaged by

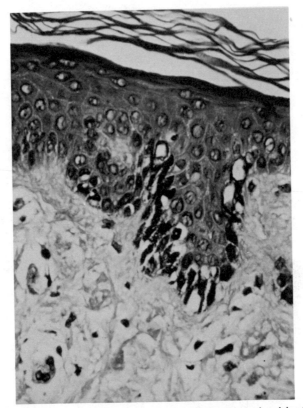

Fig 4–5.—Epidermal basal cells in darkly pigmented subject, showing marked cytoplasmic vacuolization and nuclear pyknosis after laser treatment.

pulsed tunable dye lasers opens the prospect of improving the laser treatment of vascular lesions of the skin, such as port-wine hemangiomas. While argon laser therapy is efficacious in most cases, the cosmetic result is marred by excessive scarring in up to 15% of patients. Epidermal damage and cicatrization may be decreased by laser protocols that use optic targeting of hemoglobin. Port-wine hemangiomas have been successfully treated with a continuous-wave dye laser tuned to 540 nm (the β band of oxyhemoglobin). No epidermal damage occurred following a 100 to 200 msec exposure,

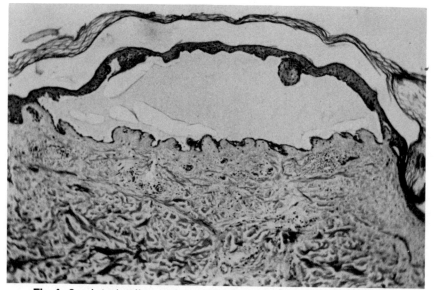

Fig 4–6.—Intrabasilar vesicle following pulsed laser irradiation of darkly pigmented subject. Clinical purpura was not detected, but vascular damage was present histologically, in addition to epidermal changes.

whereas comparable doses of the argon laser caused extensive dermal and epidermal damage.

Pulsed dye lasers tuned to 577 nm have also been used to treat port-wine hemangioma with variable results. One group reported good clinical results following serial monthly treatments, each of which consisted of a 0.7-μsec pulse of up to 70 joules/cm^2. Another group had no success using a single 0.6-μsec pulse of 3 joules/cm^2; in this case, there may have been such well-confined vascular damage that the host's fibrotic response was inadequate to compress the ectatic vessels and thereby effect a good cosmetic result. More studies with dye lasers are needed to establish the optimal parameters of dose, pulse duration, and histologic end points required to clear port-wine hemangiomas without causing unnecessary damage to other structures, such as the epidermis.

Quite a different application of tunable dye lasers is in the photodynamic therapy of cancers, using human hematoporphyrin derivative (HPD). In photodynamic therapy, continuous-wave laser irradiation causes the nonthermal, photochemical destruction of cancer cells, which selectively retain the HPD. While the mechanism of HPD photodynamic therapy is primarily photochemical, the irradiation of sensitized skin also causes a temperature rise of up to 7 C; this localized hyperthermia acts synergistically with the photochemical mechanism to control experimental tumors. The temperature rise associated with continuous-wave photodynamic therapy is far below that found with high-power pulsed laser therapy. This treatment method generally uses an argon laser to pump the dye laser, which is tuned to 630 nm, a wavelength that corresponds to a minor absorbance peak of HPD that produces reasonably deep penetration into tissue. Alternatively, a helium-neon (HeNe) laser (at 633 nm) or a gold vapor laser (at 628 nm) can be used.

In dermatology, this approach has been used to treat squamous cell carcinoma, melanoma, Kaposi's sarcoma, Bowen's disease, basal cell carcinoma, and metastatic breast carcinoma. Favorable results have been reported, and research on this experimental cancer therapy continues. HPD photodynamic therapy may also be effective in psoriasis and in other benign hyperproliferative diseases. The formulation of topical HPD preparations may make this approach to nonmalignant skin disease more acceptable. The results are preliminary, however, and more work is needed. The main side effect of HPD photodynamic therapy is the photosensitization of normal skin, because HPD has only partial selectivity for cancer cells. This technique is likely to prove more valuable when the active therapeutic components of HPD have been better isolated and purified and when a means for more specific localization to tumors has been discovered.

COPPER VAPOR LASER

Studies with the copper vapor laser were prompted by observations on the selective vascular effects of 300-nsec pulses of the dye laser tuned to 577 nm. The copper vapor laser was chosen because its wavelength of 578 nm is virtually the same as that of the tunable dye laser. The continuous train of micropulses (30-nsec pulses at 5 kHz) could be gated to achieve macropulses that delivered biologically effective doses in 4 to 60 msec. Pulse duration could thus be studied as an independent variable. (The results suggest that the biologic responses to the micropulses are additive, but this finding needs to be confirmed.)

Ten fair-skinned white volunteers were exposed to a dose ranging from 1 to 30 joules/cm^2 at an average power density of either 1,300 or 4,000 W/cm^2, and their skin was examined grossly and by biopsy. At threshold doses, copper vapor laser exposure caused immediate pain, erythema, and opacification of the skin surface. Purpura, the hallmark response to 300-nsec pulsed radiation, never occurred with the longer-pulsed source; conversely, opacification did not occur at any dose level with 300-nsec pulses. The average thresholds for both opacification and delayed erythema were slightly but significantly lower when the higher power density was used. In no subject was the lower power density more efficient in producing delayed erythema or opacification.

Histologically, at the threshold doses for gross changes there was a variable degree of basal epidermal necrosis. Dermal changes included endothelial swelling and necrosis, loss of polarization in Masson's trichrome—stained sections, and fibrin deposition. At doses above the threshold level, full-thickness epidermal necrosis as well as deeper dermal collagen denaturation and hemorrhage were often noted.

These histologic findings can be contrasted with the specific vascular effects of the 577-nm tunable dye laser at pulse durations ranging from 300 nsec to 400 msec. The differences between the two methods arise from the premise that the thermal energy that is initially deposited at the absorbing blood pigments is diffused more widely into surrounding structures when longer pulsewidths (such as those of the copper vapor laser) are used. The absence of gross purpura or microscopic hemorrhage at threshold doses with the copper vapor laser may signify that heating with pulsewidths of tens of milliseconds does not involve rapid expansion or microvaporization of blood. The opacification presumably represents protein denaturation. These studies serve to emphasize that pulse duration is an important determinant of biologic response, independent of wavelength.

The threshold doses for gross skin damage by the copper vapor laser are similar to those required with the argon laser, at 200 msec (a long time compared to the time required to heat tissue around vessels and injure the entire exposed field). The finding that higher power densities (with correspondingly shorter exposure times of 5 to 10 msec) caused a lowering of the threshold dose suggests that at shorter pulse durations equal amounts of perivascular and endothelial cell injury may occur with less total energy. This proposed relationship supports theoretical calculations that the thermal relaxation time of cutaneous vessels is in the millisecond range.

ULTRAVIOLET EXCIMER LASERS

The active medium in these instruments is a combination of a rare gas with a halide; either a halide-oxide or a halide-halide dimer can be used. These dimeric mediums are excited to emit pulsed laser radiation, hence the name excited dimer, or excimer. Depending on the chemical composition of the medium, different ultraviolet wavelengths are emitted (Table 4–2).

High-power excimer lasers are used to ablate organic polymers in thin layers; the mechanism is unclear. Very high temperatures are reached in microscopic volumes, so thermal mechanisms are probably involved. Photochemical disruption of bonds may also occur, however; the photoproducts may be volatile or unstable, leading to ablation. The laser would thus act as a "photochemical knife."

Excimer lasers have been used to ablate tissues, including cornea and artery. Unlike CO_2 laser energy, which is absorbed by water, the major biologic target of ultraviolet excimer lasers is protein. Lane and colleagues ablated human and guinea pig skin in vitro and guinea pig skin in vivo, using a 14-nsec pulsed excimer laser em-

TABLE 4–2.—ULTRAVIOLET EXCIMER
LASER

ACTIVE MEDIUM	WAVELENGTH (NM)
Fluoride (F_2)	157
Argon fluoride (ArF)	193
Krypton fluoride (KrF)	248
Xenon chloride (XeCl)	308
Xenon fluoride (XeF)	351

ploying argon fluoride and krypton fluoride with a pulse repetition rate of up to 4.7 cycles/second. They created clean-edged incisions in excised guinea pig skin by irradiating it with graded fluences at either 193 nm or 248 nm delivered in a beam 1 mm in diameter. Electron micrographs of collagen fibrils show a zone of damage confined to within 100 μm of the ablative surface. The depth of incision is a direct function of the number of pulses delivered. With a wavelength of 193 nm, about 1.0 μm of tissue was ablated per pulse, independent of power density; with a wavelength of 248 nm, however, the depth of ablation was a strongly positive function of power density. With either wavelength, the rate of ablation was similar in the different layers of guinea pig skin. Human skin irradiated in vitro showed similar precise, thermally confined damage. But the rate of ablation of human skin was fluence dependent for both the 193-nm and the 248-nm wavelength.

Irradiation of guinea pig skin in vivo at 193 nm caused the ablation to extend to the papillary dermis, with the depth of ablation a function of the exposure dose. When ablation proceeded to the depth of the dermal vessels, however, and bleeding started, further exposure did not cause deeper ablation; instead, collagen denaturation extended farther laterally into the surrounding tissue (250 μm). Irradiation at 248 nm, in contrast, caused deeper extension of ablation into the subcutaneous tissues despite bleeding.

This study was important in that it demonstrated the practicability of ablation of skin by ultraviolet excimer laser radiation and in that it confirmed the extreme spatial confinement of the thermal effects of this method. The study also underscored the dependence of ablation on wavelength and the importance of testing in vitro results in well-chosen in vivo experiments.

Future clinical dermatologic applications of these tools may include ablation of benign new growths and nevi and certain plastic surgery procedures. As a research tool, ultrathin ablation provides a more controlled method than cellophane tape stripping for studies of stratum corneum function and percutaneous absorption.

The issue of carcinogenicity must be addressed before ultraviolet excimer laser treatments can be widely applied. Mutagenesis has been demonstrated at most ultraviolet wavelengths. The action spectra for mutagenesis and carcinogenesis are similar to that for erythema, indicating that similar chromophores (e.g., DNA) may

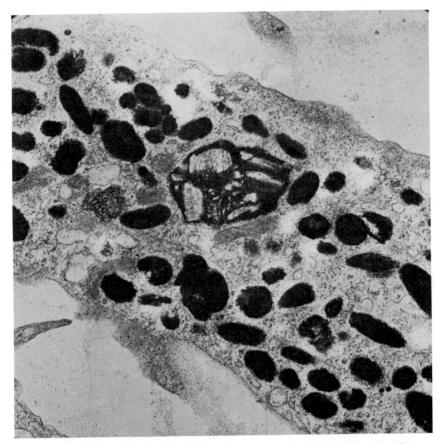

Fig 4–7.—High-power view of an aberrant melanosome following ultraviolet irradiation of melanocyte in vitro.

initiate both pathways. The carcinogenicity of the 254-nm wavelength is particularly well documented, because of the availability of the 254-nm emission line of the mercury vapor lamp. The carcinogenicity and other biologic effects of the 193-nm wavelength are not well studied. Wavelengths that are less than 200 nm are expected to cause the formation of different photoproducts in DNA and other biomolecules than wavelengths that are greater than 200 nm.

It is likely that these short-wave ultraviolet energies will prove to be mutagenic and carcinogenic, although it is not clear what such a finding implies for therapy. Many current applications of phototherapy use carcinogenic wavelengths, for example, psoralen ultraviolet-A (PUVA) photochemotherapy and UV-B phototherapy of psoriasis. The risk/benefit ratio must be decided in each case.

Ultraviolet excimer lasers have also been used in subablative energy densities for research. Human epidermal melanocyte cultures irradiated at doses greater than 0.1 joule/cm^2 were extensively damaged within one hour of exposure to the ultraviolet excimer laser at the 351-nm wavelength given in 20-nsec pulses (Fig 4–7). When nonpigmented cells, comprising cultures of normal human dermal fibroblasts and human bladder tumor cell lines, were treated under the same conditions, they remained unaltered. Irradiation of human skin in vivo with 10-nsec pulses at 351 nm caused selective damage to melanosomes within melanocytes and keratinocytes, without causing damage to nuclei, mitochondria, and so on. These results show that selective photothermolysis at the organelle level can be carried out with unfocused laser light on millions of cells simultaneously in vivo to produce a form of in vivo microsurgery. Future clinical applications may include the treatment of benign pigmented tissues.

A PERSPECTIVE ON LASER PHOTOMEDICINE

This survey shows a trend in laser photomedicine. The laser was, of course, recognized as an optic instrument in its earliest applications, but the main variables that were then being manipulated were simply power and delivered energy. These early instruments offered little versatility with respect to wavelength and pulse duration, and their application was not predicated on any detailed model of tissue optics. As new lasers became available, new medical applications were found for them, through a process of trial and error.

In recent years, tissue optics has been recognized as important for research and development in laser therapeutics. The detailed optics of normal skin and other tissues is still problematic; the optics of diseased tissue is even less well characterized. We expect that major advances in laser photomedicine will stem from a better understanding and refined manipulation of tissue optics. As this change happens, we expect to see a greater rapprochement between laser surgery and photobiology. Historically, these two fields have been curiously separated, probably because the unique properties of lasers may lead workers in this area to regard research on the more conventional light sources as less exciting. For their part, photochemists and photobiologists have generally viewed heating by light, which is a common result of high-power laser irradiation, as an experimental side effect to be avoided.

This dichotomy between lasers and other light sources reflects an important difference in the mechanisms by which particular instruments can be used for selective therapeutic effects. Most forms of phototherapy or photochemotherapy result from in vivo photochemistry. The factors that determine how the light is selectively absorbed to provide more benefits than risks are therefore at the molecular level, intrinsic to the resulting chemical reactions. In these treatment methods, the biologic responses depend on the total number of photons absorbed, not on the intensity of the light source. Because large areas of the body must usually be treated, conventional light sources are acceptable and are, in fact, required for therapy in most cases. Ultraviolet radiation treatment of psoriasis and blue-light phototherapy of hyperbilirubinemia of newborn infants are good examples of phototherapy. Photodynamic treatment of tumors with HPD and lasers is also based on photochemistry; the selectivity in this approach comes from confining specific chemical reactions to the HPD-targeted cells.

Most laser therapy, however, depends on thermal mechanisms; in this case, the effects are dependent on the intensity of the laser light. Selectivity with lasers usually results from the spatial confinement of heat. Lasers are used to cook, boil, explode, vaporize, or ablate very small volumes of tissue. Spatial confinement of a focused beam to a small volume of tissue may lead to therapies that depend on the thermal denaturation of macromolecules, resulting in cell death and focal coagulation necrosis. Cutting and ablating applications depend on the generation of very high temperatures in very small volumes. A decrease in the total volume of denatured tissue leads to relative decreases in the host response and side effects. While this decrease in volume is usually accomplished by focusing the laser beam onto a small area, studies on selective photothermolysis show that time-resolved spatial confinement of heating can also be effected by using brief pulse durations and by exploiting the optic nonuniformities of tissue. The advantage of selective photothermolysis is that it can be used for targeting within turbid tissues, whereas the focused beam can be used only in the eye or on surface lesions.

The host responses to such "internal heating" are largely unknown. It is only with the advent of lasers that this type of biologic experiment has been possible. Over the millions of years of organic evolution, specific mechanisms of repair for such damage have therefore not been developed. In contrast, mechanisms of repair exist for damage produced by ultraviolet and ionizing radiation and by other forms of thermal stress that occur in natural states.

The versatility of selective photothermolysis will be greatly enhanced if suitable exogenous chromophores can be administered selectively to targets of choice, such as tumors, bleeding lesions, and atheromatous plaques. One approach to selective targeting is to bond chromophores to monoclonal antibodies; alternatively, chemical affinity might be exploited (consider, for example, the affinity of many tumor cells for dyes such as HPD and acridine orange). Unlike targeted therapy with toxins or radionuclides, laser photochemotherapy relies on the synergism between light and drug, which diminishes the toxicity to nonirradiated body areas that may also concentrate the drug.

The photochemical properties that would be desirable in chromophores used in selective photothermolysis may differ from those of photochemical toxins such as HPD. These thermogenic dyes ideally would be both thermally stable and photostable, so as to permit repeated photon absorptions during irradiation. While fluorescence is a useful diagnostic property in biologic dyes, in that it permits localization and quantification within targets, very high fluorescence quantum efficiency may be a disadvantage in dyes that are intended to convert almost all of the absorbed energy into heat. For both classes of dyes, the optical absorbance should be high within the therapeutic window between 600 and 1,200 nm, so as to minimize competition by endogenous pigments.

It is conceivable that the optics of skin could be creatively modified by laser irradiation itself. For instance, one laser, perhaps in combination with a drug, might be used to prime the tissue optically for therapeutic irradiation by another laser. The effect of laser irradiation on skin optics is almost unstudied, but clearly an alteration thus produced could affect both the biologic response and the optical measurements of that response (e.g., by remittance spectroscopy). Conversely, studies of the optical effects of laser irradiation may provide a new direction for research and may give insight into the basic mechanisms of laser-tissue interactions. In the future, we may have instruments that simultaneously irradiate tissue and take optical measurements of the field ("smart lasers"). Such tools could be programmed by computer to vary the wavelength, pulse duration, and irradiance in response to the changing optics of the target; for instance, the laser would automatically go into the hemostasis mode when hemoglobin was detected by remittance data. By this means, the ratio of cutting to sealing could be continuously optimized for different procedures. Eventually, computers may also be used to gate laser pulses to a certain point in the cardiac cycle during laser angioplasty of the coronary arteries.

Medical applications of lasers have been increasing because of the same unique properties that have made them important tools for materials processing. The spatial coherence and attendant collimation of laser beams allow focusing to spot sizes on the order of the optical wavelength and provide the high intensities needed for spatially localized heating. Beam collimation allows convenient manipulation by optical systems such as articulated arms. The variety of high-power laser sources available, spanning the region from ultraviolet to infrared, makes it possible to produce power densities that could not be produced with conventional sources. In biomedical applications, however, materials processing (e.g., physical change or treatment) is only the first step; the host response completes the treatment, and in many cases this response is the paramount determinant of the final result. Manipulation of host responses to laser irradiation may become the key to new therapies.

Another possible application of lasers someday might be to initiate photochemical reactions that either activate a drug, deactivate it, or alter its disposition (e.g., release it from a photolabile liposome). Such a "photopharmaceutical" drug could act by many different mechanisms, with the photochemical event modifying only the pharmacokinetics. This mode of action is in contrast to that of classical photochemotherapy (e.g., with PUVA or HPD), in which the photochemical event itself represents the crucial pharmacologic step. One can even envision a photochemical cascade (laser emission, absorption of photons by tissue or photopharmaceutical, fluorescence, absorption of the fluoresced photon by another chromophore, etc.) by which an amplified photopharmaceutical response could occur. When this possibility becomes an actuality, nonsurgical laser medicine will truly have come of age.

Already a valuable surgical tool, the laser in medicine is evolving to include diagnostic and pharmacologic uses that may eventually prove equally important. We expect that the skin, because of its unique position as the interface between the organism and its environment, will continue to be studied as a model for these laser-tissue interactions, and that clinical dermatology will continue to be an important arena for new advances in laser phototherapy.

BIBLIOGRAPHY

Abergel, R. P., et al. Laser treatment of keloids. *Lasers Surg. Med.* 4:291–295, 1984.

Abergel, R. P., et al. Nonthermal effects of Nd:YAG laser on biological functions of human skin fibroblasts in culture. *Lasers Surg. Med.* 3:279–284, 1984.

Anderson, R. R., and Parrish, J. A. Microvasculature can be selectively damaged using dye lasers: a basic theory and experimental evidence in human skin. *Lasers Surg. Med.* 1:263–276, 1981.

Anderson, R. R., and Parrish, J. A. The optics of human skin. *J. Invest. Dermatol.* 77:13–19, 1981.

Anderson, R. R., and Parrish, J. A. Selective photothermolysis: precise microsurgery by selective absorption of pulsed radiation. *Science* 220:524–527, 1983.

Anderson, R. R.; Harrist, T. J.; and Parrish, J. A. Unpublished observations.

Anderson, R. R.; Jaenicke, K. F.; and Parrish, J. A. Mechanisms of selective vascular changes by dye lasers. *Lasers Surg. Med.* 3:211–215, 1983.

Bandieramonte, G., et al. Hematoporphyrin-derivative and phototherapy in extensive basal-cell carcinoma of the dorsal skin. In *Porphyrins in tumor phototherapy,* ed. A. Andreoni and R. Cubedder. New York: Plenum, 1984, pp. 389–394.

Berns, M. W., et al. Response of psoriasis to red laser light (630nm) following systemic injection of hematoporphyrin derivative. *Lasers Surg. Med.* 4:73–77, 1984.

Berns, M. W.; Coffey, J.; and Wile, A. G. Laser photoradiation therapy of cancer: possible role of hyperthermia. *Lasers Surg. Med.* 4:87–92, 1984.

Castro, D. J., et al. Wound healing: biological effects of Nd:YAG laser on collagen metabolism in pig skin in comparison to thermal burn. *Ann. Plast. Surg.* 11:131–140, 1983.

Diette, K. M.; Bronstein, B. R.; and Parrish, J. A. Histologic comparison of argon and tunable dye lasers in the treatment of tattoos. In press.

Dixon, J. A. Argon laser treatment of port wine stains. In *Cutaneous laser therapy*, ed. K. A. Arndt, J. M. Noe, and S. Rosen. New York: John Wiley & Sons, 1983, pp. 109–128.

Dougherty, T. J. Photoradiation therapy for cutaneous and subcutaneous malignancies. *J. Invest. Dermatol.* 77:122–124, 1981.

Dougherty, T. J.; Boyle, D. G.; and Weishaupt, K. R. Photoradiation therapy of human tumors. In *The science of photomedicine*, ed. J. D. Regan and J. A. Parrish. New York: Plenum, 1982, pp. 625–637.

Gange, R. W., et al. Effect of pre-irradiation tissue target temperature upon selective vascular damage induced by 577 nm tunable dye laser pulses. *Microvasc. Res.* 28:125–130, 1984.

Garcia, R. I., et al. Effects of ultraviolet excimer laser radiation on human melanocyte cultures. In *Proceedings of the International Pigment Cell Conference, Pigment Cell*, Vol. 7, in press.

Gardner, W. N., et al. Quantitative analysis of effect of neodymium-YAG laser on transplanted mouse carcinomas. *Thorax* 37:594–597, 1982.

Goldman, J.; Hornby, P.; and Long, C. Effect of the laser on the skin. III. Transmission of laser beams through fiber optics. *J. Invest. Dermatol.* 42:231–234, 1964.

Goldman, L. Comparison of the biomedical effects of the exposure of human tissues to low and high energy lasers. *Ann. N.Y. Acad. Sci.* 122:802–831, 1965.

Goldman, L. Laser surgery for skin cancer. *N.Y. State J. Med.* 77:1897–1900, 1977.

Goldman, L. Surgery by laser for malignant melanoma. *J. Dermatol. Surg. Oncol.* 5:141–144, 1979.

Goldman, L., et al. Radiation from a Q-switched ruby laser. *J. Invest. Dermatol.* 44:69–71, 1965.

Goldman, L., et al. Effect of the laser beam on the skin. *J. Invest. Dermatol.* 40:121–122, 1963.

Goldman, L., et al. High-power neodymium-YAG laser surgery. *Acta Derm. Venereol.* (Stockh.) 53:45–49, 1973.

Goldman, L., et al. Laser radiation of malignancy in man. *Cancer* 18:533–545, 1965.

Goldman, L., et al. Pathology of the effect of the laser beam on the skin. *Nature* 197:912–914, 1963.

Goldman, L., and Dreffer, R. Laser treatment of extensive mixed cavernous and port-wine stains. *Arch. Dermatol.* 113:504–505, 1977.

Goldman, L.; Igelman, J. M.; and Richfield, D. F. Impact of the laser on nevi and melanomas. *Arch. Dermatol.* 90:71–75, 1964.

Goldman, L.; Siler, V. E., and Blaney, D. Laser therapy of melanomas. *Surg. Gynecol. Obstet.* 124:49–56, 1967.

Greenwald, J., et al. Comparative histologic studies of the tunable dye (at 577 nm) laser and argon laser: the specific vascular effects of the dye laser. *J. Invest. Dermatol.* 77:305–310, 1981.

Helsper, J. T., et al. The biological effect of laser energy on human melanoma. *Cancer* 17:1299–1304, 1964.

Henderson, D. L., et al. Argon and carbon dioxide laser treatment of hypertrophic and keloid scars. *Lasers Surg. Med.* 3:271–277, 1984.

Hoye, R. C.; Ketcham, A. S.; and Riggle, G. C. The air-borne dissemination of viable tumor by high-energy neodymium laser. *Life Sci.* 6:119–125, 1967.

Hulsbergen Henning, J. P., et al. Experimental treatment of port wine stain haemangioma with a 577 nm pulsed dye laser. Presented at the Fifth International Congress of Laser Medicine and Surgery, September 1983, Detroit.

Hulsbergen Henning, J. P., and Van Gemert, M. J. C. Port wine stain coagulation experiments with a 540-nm continuous wave dye-laser. *Lasers Surg. Med.* 2:205–210, 1983.

Konaka, C., and Ono, J. Skin metastases from breast cancer. In *Lasers and hematoporphyrin derivative in cancer,* ed. Y. Hayata and T. J. Dougherty, transl. J. P. Banon. New York: Igaku-Shoin, 1983, pp. 110–114.

Kozlov, A. P., et al. Antitumor effect of laser radiation. *Acta Radiol.* [Diagn.] (Stockh.) 12:241–256, 1973.

Kozlov, A. P., and Moskalik, K. G. Pulsed laser radiation therapy of skin tumors. *Cancer* 46:2172–2178, 1980.

Lane, R. J.; Linsker, R.; and Wynne, J. J. Ultraviolet-laser ablation of skin. *Lasers Surg. Med.,* in press.

Laub, D. R., et al. Preliminary histopathological observation of Q-switched ruby laser irradiation of dermal tattoo pigment in man. *J. Surg. Res.* 8:220–224, 1968.

Linsker, R., et al. Far-ultraviolet ablation of atherosclerotic lesions. *Lasers Surg. Med.* 4:201–206, 1984.

McCullough, J. L., et al. Development of a topical hematoporphyrin derivative formulation. *J. Invest. Dermatol.* 81:528–532, 1983.

McGuff, P. E.; Deterling, R. A.; and Gottlieb, L. S. Laser radiation for metastatic malignant melanoma. *J.A.M.A.* 195:393–394, 1966.

McGuff, P. E.; Deterling, R. A.; and Gottlieb, L. S. Tumoricidal effect of laser energy on experimental and human malignant tumors. *N. Engl. J. Med.* 273:490–492, 1965.

Minton, J. P., et al. An evaluation of the physical response of malignant tumor implants to pulsed laser radiation. *Surg. Gynecol. Obstet.* 120:538–544, 1965.

Murphy, G. F., et al. Organelle-specific injury to melanin-containing cells in human skin by pulsed laser irradiation. *Lab. Invest.* 49:680–685, 1983.

Ohshiro, T., et al. Le laser à l'argon et le laser au rubis dans le traitement des taches cutanées pigmentées. *Ann. Chir. Plast.* 26:231–236, 1981.

Ohshiro, T., et al. Treatment of pigmentation of the lips and oral mucosa in Peutz-Jeghers' syndrome using ruby and argon lasers. *Br. J. Plast. Surg.* 33:346–349, 1980.

Ohshiro, T., and Maruyama, Y. The ruby and argon lasers in the treatment of naevi. *Ann. Acad. Med. Singapore* 12:388–395, 1983.

Oseroff, A. R., et al. Dye-enhancement and pulsewidth dependence of selective laser-induced thermal injury to cutaneous vessels. *J. Invest. Dermatol.* (abstr.) 82:435, 1984.

Parrish, J. A. New concepts in therapeutic photomedicine: photochemistry, optical targeting and the therapeutic window. *J. Invest. Dermatol.* 77:45–50, 1981.

Parrish, J. A., et al. Cutaneous effects of pulsed nitrogen gas laser irradiation. *J. Invest. Dermatol.* 67:603–68, 1976.

Parrish, J. A., et al. Selective thermal effects with pulsed irradiation from lasers: from organ to organelle. *J. Invest. Dermatol.* 80(suppl.):75S–80S, 1983.

Paul, B. S., et al. The effect of temperature and other factors on selective microvascular damage caused by pulsed dye laser. *J. Invest. Dermatol.* 81:333–335, 1983.

Reid, W. H., et al. Q-switched ruby laser treatment of black tattoos. *Br. J. Plast. Surg.* 36:455–459, 1983.

Soloman, H., et al. Histopathology of the laser treatment of portwine lesions. *J. Invest. Dermatol.* 50:141–146, 1968.

Tan, O. T.; Kerschmann, R.; and Parrish, J. A. The effect of epidermal pigmentation on selective vascular effects of pulsed laser. *Lasers Surg. Med.*, in press, 1984.

Tokuda, Y. Primary skin cancer. In *Lasers and hematoporphyrin derivative in cancer*, ed. Y. Hayata and T. J. Dougherty, transl. J. P. Barron, New York: Igaku-Shoin, 1983, pp. 88–96.

Trokel, S.; Srivasan, R.; and Braren, B. Laser surgery of the cornea. *Am. J. Ophthalmol.* 96:710–715, 1983.

Urbach, F. Photocarcinogenesis. In *The science of photomedicine*, ed. J. D. Regan and J. A. Parrish. New York: Plenum, 1982, pp. 261–292.

Wagner, R. I., et al. Laser therapy of human benign and malignant neoplasms of the skin. *Acta Radiol.* [Diagn.] (Stockh.) 14:417–423, 1975.

Wagner, R. I.; Kozlov, A. P.; and Moskalik, K. G. Laser radiation therapy of skin melanoma. *Strahlentherapie* 157:670–672, 1981.

Wakamatsu, S.; Hirayama, T.; and Takahashi, K. Dye laser system and its application to port wine stains. Presented at the Fifth International Congress of Laser Medicine and Surgery, September 1983, Detroit.

Waldow, S. M.; Henderson, B. W.; and Dougherty, T. J. Enhanced tumor control following sequential treatments of photodynamic therapy (PDT) and localized microwave hyperthermia in vivo. *Lasers Surg. Med.* 4:79–85, 1984.

Wan, S.; Anderson, R. R.; and Parrish, J. A. Analytical modeling for the optical properties of the skin with *in vitro* and *in vivo* applications. *Photochem. Photobiol.* 34:493–499, 1981.

Yules, R. B., et al. The effect of Q-switched ruby laser radiation on dermal tattoo pigment in man. *Arch. Surg.* 95:179–180, 1967.

Zorat, P. L., et al. Hematoporphyrin phototherapy of malignant tumors. In *Porphyrins in tumor phototherapy*, ed. A. Andreoni and R. Cubedder. New York: Plenum, 1984, pp. 381–387.

INDEX

133